T0362328

Controversies of the Anterolateral Complex of the Knee

Editors

FREDDIE H. FU
MARCIN KOWALCZUK

CLINICS IN
SPORTS MEDICINE

www.sportsmed.theclinics.com

Consulting Editor
MARK D. MILLER

January 2018 • Volume 37 • Number 1

ELSEVIER

1600 John F. Kennedy Boulevard ● Suite 1800 ● Philadelphia, Pennsylvania, 19103-2899

http://www.theclinics.com

CLINICS IN SPORTS MEDICINE Volume 37, Number 1
January 2018 ISSN 0278-5919, ISBN-13: 978-0-323-56657-5

Editor: Lauren Boyle
Developmental Editor: Donald Mumford

© **2018 Elsevier Inc. All rights reserved.**

This periodical and the individual contributions contained in it are protected under copyright by Elsevier, and the following terms and conditions apply to their use:

Photocopying

Single photocopies of single articles may be made for personal use as allowed by national copyright laws. Permission of the Publisher and payment of a fee is required for all other photocopying, including multiple or systematic copying, copying for advertising or promotional purposes, resale, and all forms of document delivery. Special rates are available for educational institutions that wish to make photocopies for non-profit educational classroom use. For information on how to seek permission visit www.elsevier.com/permissions or call: (+44) 1865 843830 (UK)/(+1) 215 239 3804 (USA).

Derivative Works

Subscribers may reproduce tables of contents or prepare lists of articles including abstracts for internal circulation within their institutions. Permission of the Publisher is required for resale or distribution outside the institution. Permission of the Publisher is required for all other derivative works, including compilations and translations (please consult www.elsevier.com/permissions).

Electronic Storage or Usage

Permission of the Publisher is required to store or use electronically any material contained in this periodical, including any article or part of an article (please consult www.elsevier.com/permissions). Except as outlined above, no part of this publication may be reproduced, stored in a retrieval system or transmitted in any form or by any means, electronic, mechanical, photocopying, recording or otherwise, without prior written permission of the Publisher.

Notice

No responsibility is assumed by the Publisher for any injury and/or damage to persons or property as a matter of products liability, negligence or otherwise, or from any use or operation of any methods, products, instructions or ideas contained in the material herein. Because of rapid advances in the medical sciences, in particular, independent verification of diagnoses and drug dosages should be made.

Although all advertising material is expected to conform to ethical (medical) standards, inclusion in this publication does not constitute a guarantee or endorsement of the quality or value of such product or of the claims made of it by its manufacturer.

Clinics in Sports Medicine (ISSN 0278-5919) is published quarterly by Elsevier Inc., 360 Park Avenue South, New York, NY 10010-1710. Months of issue are January, April, July, and October. Business and Editorial Offices: 1600 John F. Kennedy Blvd., Ste. 1800, Philadelphia, PA 19103-2899. Customer Service Office: 3251 Riverport Lane, Maryland Heights, MO 63043. Periodicals postage paid at New York, NY and additional mailing offices. Subscription prices are $357.00 per year (US individuals), $664.00 per year (US institutions), $100.00 per year (US students), $405.00 per year (Canadian individuals), $820.00 per year (Canadian institutions), $235.00 (Canadian students), $475.00 per year (foreign individuals), $820.00 per year (foreign institutions), and $235.00 per year (foreign students). Foreign air speed delivery is included in all *Clinics* subscription prices. All prices are subject to change without notice. **POSTMASTER:** Send address changes to *Clinics in Sports Medicine*, Elsevier Health Sciences Division, Subscription Customer Service, 3251 Riverport Lane, Maryland Heights, MO 63043. Customer Service (orders, claims, online, change of address): Elsevier Health Sciences Division, Subscription Customer Service, 3251 Riverport Lane, Maryland Heights, MO 63043. **Tel: 1-800-654-2452 (U.S. and Canada); 314-447-8871 (outside U.S. and Canada). Fax: 314-447-8029. E-mail: journalscustomerservice-usa@elsevier.com (for print support); journalsonlinesupport-usa@ elsevier.com (for online support).**

Reprints. For copies of 100 or more of articles in this publication, please contact the Commercial Reprints Department, Elsevier Inc., 360 Park Avenue South, New York, NY 10010-1710. Tel.: 212-633-3874; Fax: 212-633-3820; E-mail: reprints@elsevier.com.

Clinics in Sports Medicine is covered in *MEDLINE/PubMed (Index Medicus) Current Contents/Clinical Medicine, Excerpta Medica,* and *ISI/Biomed.*

Contributors

CONSULTING EDITOR

MARK D. MILLER, MD
S. Ward Casscells Professor, Head, Division of Sports Medicine, Department of Orthopaedic Surgery, University of Virginia, Charlottesville, Virginia, USA; Team Physician, James Madison University, Director, Miller Review Course, Harrisonburg, Virginia, USA

EDITORS

FREDDIE H. FU, MD
Chair, Department of Orthopaedic Surgery, Distinguished Service Professor, David Silver Professor, Division of Sports Medicine, University of Pittsburgh, UPMC Sports Medicine, Pittsburgh, Pennsylvania, USA

MARCIN KOWALCZUK, MD, FRCSC
Department of Orthopaedic Surgery, University of Pittsburgh, UPMC Sports Medicine, Pittsburgh, Pennsylvania, USA

AUTHORS

MARCIO ALBERS, MD
Department of Orthopaedic Surgery, University of Pittsburgh, UPMC Sports Medicine, Pittsburgh, Pennsylvania, USA

ANDREW A. AMIS, FREng, DSc
Biomechanics Group, Mechanical Engineering Department, Imperial College London, Musculoskeletal Surgery Group, Faculty of Medicine, Charing Cross Hospital, London, United Kingdom

OLUFEMI R. AYENI, MD, MSc, FRCSC
Department of Clinical Epidemiology and Biostatistics, Centre for Evidence-Based Orthopaedics, McMaster University, McMaster University Medical Center, Hamilton, Ontario, Canada

CÉCILE BATAILLER, MD
Orthopaedic Surgery, Center Albert Trillat, Lyon North University Hospital, Lyon, France

ALICE BONDI, MD
Rizzoli-Sicilia Department, Istituto Ortopedico Rizzoli, Bagheria, Palermo, Italy

JEREMY M. BURNHAM, MD
Department of Orthopaedic Surgery, University of Pittsburgh, UPMC Sports Medicine, Pittsburgh, Pennsylvania, USA

SALVATORE CALDERONE, MD
Rizzoli-Sicilia Department, Istituto Ortopedico Rizzoli, Bagheria, Palermo, Italy

SIMONE CERCIELLO, MD
Orthopaedic Surgery, Casa di Cura Villa Betania, Rome, Italy; Orthopaedic Surgery, Marrelli Hospital, Crotone, Italy

JORGE CHAHLA, MD, PhD
Steadman Philippon Research Institute, Vail, Colorado, USA

MARK E. CINQUE, MS
Steadman Philippon Research Institute, Vail, Colorado, USA

NADER DARWICH, MD
Healthpoint, Abu Dhabi Knee & Sports Medicine Centre, Abu Dhabi, United Arab Emirates

RICHARD E. DEBSKI, PhD
Orthopaedic Robotics Laboratory, Departments of Bioengineering and Orthopaedic Surgery, University of Pittsburgh, Pittsburgh, Pennsylvania, USA

DAVID DEJOUR, MD
Orthopaedic Department, Lyon-Ortho-Clinic, Clinique de la Sauvegarde, Lyon, France

AAD DHOLLANDER, MD, PT, PhD
Clinical Fellow, Fowler Kennedy Sport Medicine Clinic, Western University, London, Ontario, Canada

ANDREW DUONG, MSc
Division of Orthopaedic Surgery, Department of Surgery, McMaster University, Hamilton, Ontario, Canada

GERALD A. FERRER, BS
Orthopaedic Robotics Laboratory, Department of Bioengineering, University of Pittsburgh, Pittsburgh, Pennsylvania, USA

FREDDIE H. FU, MD
Chair, Department of Orthopaedic Surgery, Distinguished Service Professor, David Silver Professor, Division of Sports Medicine, University of Pittsburgh, UPMC Sports Medicine, Pittsburgh, Pennsylvania, USA

ANDREW G. GEESLIN, MD
Steadman Philippon Research Institute, Vail, Colorado, USA

ALAN GETGOOD, MPhil, MD, FRCS (Tr&Orth), DipSEM
Assistant Professor, Consultant Orthopaedic Surgeon, Complex Knee Reconstruction, Fowler Kennedy Sport Medicine Clinic, Western University, London, Ontario, Canada

ALBERTO GRASSI, MD
2nd Orthopaedic and Traumatologic Clinic, Laboratory of Biomechanics and Technology Innovation, Istituto Ortopedico Rizzoli, Bologna, Italy

DANIEL GUENTHER, MD
Trauma Department, Hannover Medical School, Hannover, Germany

ELMAR HERBST, MD
Orthopaedic Robotics Laboratory, Department of Orthopaedic Surgery, University of Pittsburgh, UPMC Sports Medicine, Pittsburgh, Pennsylvania, USA; Department of Orthopaedic Sports Medicine, Klinikum rechts der Isar, Technical University Munich, Munich, Germany

NOLAN S. HORNER, MD
Department of Medicine, Michael G. DeGroote School of Medicine, McMaster University, Hamilton, Ontario, Canada

EIVIND INDERHAUG, MD, MPH, PhD
Orthopaedic Surgery Department, Surgical Clinic, Haraldsplass Deaconess Hospital, Bergen, Norway; Imperial College London, London, United Kingdom

LAITH M. JAZRAWI, MD
Chief of Sports Medicine Division, NYU Langone Medical Center, New York, New York, USA

DANIEL JAMES KAPLAN, BA
Department of Orthopaedic Surgery, NYU Langone Medical Center, New York, New York, USA

CHRISTOPH KITTL, MD
Department of Trauma, Hand and Reconstructive Surgery, University of Munster, Muenster, Germany

MARCIN KOWALCZUK, MD, FRCSC
Department of Orthopaedic Surgery, University of Pittsburgh, UPMC Sports Medicine, Pittsburgh, Pennsylvania, USA

DREW LANSDOWN, MD
Assistant Professor in Residence, Department of Orthopaedic Surgery, University of California San Francisco, San Francisco, California, USA

ROBERT F. LaPRADE, MD, PhD
Steadman Philippon Research Institute, The Steadman Clinic, Vail, Colorado, USA

CHUNBONG BENJAMIN MA, MD
Professor, Department of Orthopaedic Surgery, University of California San Francisco, San Francisco, California, USA

GIULIO MARIA MARCHEGGIANI MUCCIOLI, MD
2nd Orthopaedic and Traumatologic Clinic, Laboratory of Biomechanics and Technology Innovation, Istituto Ortopedico Rizzoli, Bologna, Italy

MANOJ MATHEW, MS(ortho), FRACS
Clinical Fellow, Fowler Kennedy Sport Medicine Clinic, Western University, London, Ontario, Canada

THOMAS K. MILLER, MD
Vice Chairman and Section Chief of Sports Medicine, Carilion Clinic, Associate Professor, Department of Orthopaedic Surgery, Virginia Tech Carilion School of Medicine, Institute for Orthopaedics and Neurosciences, Roanoke, Virginia, USA

PAUL A. MOROZ, MD (Cand)
Faculty of Medicine, The University of British Columbia, Vancouver, British Columbia, Canada

VOLKER MUSAHL, MD
Orthopaedic Robotics Laboratory, Associate Professor, Departments of Bioengineering and Orthopaedic Surgery, Medical Director, UPMC Rooney Sports Complex, UPMC Sports Medicine, Program Director, Sports Medicine Fellowship, University of Pittsburgh, Pittsburgh, Pennsylvania, USA

KANTO NAGAI, MD, PhD
Orthopaedic Robotics Laboratory, Department of Orthopaedic Surgery, University of Pittsburgh, Pittsburgh, Pennsylvania, USA

PHILIPPE NEYRET, MD, PhD
Healthpoint, Abu Dhabi Knee & Sports Medicine Centre, Abu Dhabi, United Arab Emirates

PANAGIOTIS NTAGIOPOULOS, MD, PhD
Hip and Knee Unit, Mediterraneo Hospital, Athens, Greece

THIERRY PAUYO, MD, FRCSC
Department of Orthopaedic Surgery, University of Pittsburgh, UPMC Sports Medicine, Pittsburgh, Pennsylvania, USA

EMILY E. QUICK, MD (Cand)
Department of Medicine, Michael G. DeGroote School of Medicine, McMaster University, Hamilton, Ontario, Canada

FEDERICO RAGGI, MD
2nd Orthopaedic and Traumatologic Clinic, Laboratory of Biomechanics and Technology Innovation, Istituto Ortopedico Rizzoli, Bologna, Italy

MATTEO ROMAGNOLI, MD
Rizzoli-Sicilia Department, Istituto Ortopedico Rizzoli, Bagheria, Palermo, Italy

CECILIA SIGNORELLI, PhD
Laboratory of Biomechanics and Technology Innovation, Istituto Ortopedico Rizzoli, Bologna, Italy

NICOLE SIMUNOVIC, MSc
Department of Clinical Epidemiology and Biostatistics, Centre for Evidence-Based Orthopaedics, McMaster University, Hamilton, Ontario, Canada

ANDY WILLIAMS, FRCS(Orth), FFSEM
Imperial College London, Fortius Clinic, London, United Kingdom

STEFANO ZAFFAGNINI, MD
Professor, 2nd Orthopaedic and Traumatologic Clinic, Laboratory of Biomechanics and Technology Innovation, Istituto Ortopedico Rizzoli, Bologna, Italy

Contents

Erratum xiii

Foreword: ALL or None? xv

Mark D. Miller

Preface: Structures of the Anterolateral Knee: Why All the Confusion? xvii

Freddie H. Fu and Marcin Kowalczuk

A Layered Anatomic Description of the Anterolateral Complex of the Knee 1

Marcin Kowalczuk, Elmar Herbst, Jeremy M. Burnham, Marcio Albers,
Volker Musahl, and Freddie H. Fu

> Variability in anatomic terminology, dissection protocols, and use of em-
> balmed as opposed to fresh frozen specimens has led to the controversy
> surrounding the "anterolateral ligament of the knee." Conceptually the
> complex anatomy of the anterolateral knee is made up of the superficial,
> middle, deep, and capsulo-osseous layers of the iliotibial band. The ante-
> rolateral capsule is deep to these tissues and is directly attached to the
> lateral meniscus. These structures collectively form the anterolateral com-
> plex of the knee. The anterolateral complex in conjunction with the anterior
> cruciate ligament function to prevent anterolateral rotatory instability of the
> knee.

The Anterolateral Ligament Does Exist: An Anatomic Description 9

Stefano Zaffagnini, Alberto Grassi, Giulio Maria Marcheggiani Muccioli,
Federico Raggi, Matteo Romagnoli, Alice Bondi, Salvatore Calderone, and
Cecilia Signorelli

> The debate around the existence, anatomy, and role of the so-called ante-
> rolateral ligament of the knee represents one of the main sources of recent
> controversy among orthopedic surgeons. In the modern era of sports
> medicine, several content experts have contributed to the understanding
> of the anatomy of the anterolateral aspect of the knee. This article analyzes
> the historical, phylogenetic, anatomic, arthroscopic, and radiological evi-
> dence regarding the anterolateral ligament. The existence of the anterolat-
> eral ligament as a distinct ligamentous structure and its exact anatomic
> features are still matters of controversy and ongoing study.

Biomechanics of the Anterolateral Structures of the Knee 21

Christoph Kittl, Eivind Inderhaug, Andy Williams, and Andrew A. Amis

> This article describes the complex anatomic structures that pass across
> the lateral aspect of the knee, particularly the iliotibial tract and the under-
> lying anterolateral ligament and capsule. It provides data on their strength
> and roles in controlling tibiofemoral joint laxity and stability. These findings

are discussed in relation to surgery to repair or reconstruct the anatomic structures, or to create tenodeses with similar effect.

Biomechanical Proof for the Existence of the Anterolateral Ligament   33

Jorge Chahla, Andrew G. Geeslin, Mark E. Cinque, and Robert F. LaPrade

With the recent "description" of the anterolateral ligament (ALL) of the knee, its role in controlling rotational stability has reemerged. An improved understanding of the anatomy of the anterolateral complex of the knee has led to an expansion of the literature on the biomechanics of many structures, including the contribution of the iliotibial band and its deep (Kaplan) fibers, the capsulo-osseous layer, the ALL, and the lateral meniscal posterior root to knee stability. This article describes the primary and secondary roles of key anatomic structures at the anterolateral aspect of the knee.

Structural Properties of the Anterolateral Complex and Their Clinical Implications   41

Gerald A. Ferrer, Daniel Guenther, Thierry Pauyo, Elmar Herbst, Kanto Nagai, Richard E. Debski, and Volker Musahl

The role of the anterolateral complex of the knee in providing static and rotatory knee stability has been a source of renewed interest in the literature. Several studies have established a role of the anterolateral complex in controlling knee rotational stability. Although the objective quantification of knee kinematics and stability has been investigated, understanding of the structural properties of the anterolateral complex is evolving. This article highlights recent evidence pertaining to the structural properties of the anterolateral structures. The biomechanical evaluation of the structural properties of the anterolateral complex of the knee yielded minimal involvement in controlling knee rotational stability.

Secondary Stabilizers of Tibial Rotation in the Intact and Anterior Cruciate Ligament Deficient Knee   49

Daniel James Kaplan and Laith M. Jazrawi

The controversy regarding the existence and function of the anterolateral ligament or anterolateral complex has reinvigorated interest in rotational stability of the knee joint. This is particularly true of anterolateral rotary instability, as many patients, despite anatomic reconstruction of their anterior cruciate ligament, continue to experience instability. Many experts point toward compromised anterolateral restraints as the underlying culprit, namely, the anterolateral complex, which includes the iliotibial band, anterolateral capsule, lateral meniscus, and lateral collateral ligament. This article provides a breakdown of these structures, their function, biomechanical properties, and clinical importance, based on a thorough review of available literature.

Do We Need Extra-Articular Reconstructive Surgery?   61

Eivind Inderhaug and Andy Williams

With renewed interest in the lateral soft tissue envelope anatomy, there is also a rise in the popularity of extra-articular anterolateral procedures. There is reasonable laboratory-based evidence for additional benefit of such procedures, but clinical data are not sufficient to judge outcome in the long term for better or worse. Furthermore, the decision-making process to decide when to add an extra-articular procedure is lacking; there are no clinical tests or investigations to guide the clinician. This article presents an overview of the literature and reflections from the authors on the subject.

Anterolateral Ligament Reconstruction or Extra-Articular Tenodesis: Why and When? 75

Manoj Mathew, Aad Dhollander, and Alan Getgood

Residual rotational laxity following anterior cruciate ligament (ACL) reconstruction has been identified as significant concern in many patients, despite evolution of techniques. The expanding body of knowledge on the anatomy and biomechanics of the anterolateral soft tissue restraints in rotational control of the knee has reignited an interest in extra-articular reconstruction techniques for augmenting ACL reconstruction. Reconstruction techniques currently used can be broadly categorized as either lateral extra-articular tenodesis or reconstruction of the anterolateral ligament. In this article, we outline the relevant anatomy, biomechanics, and rationale behind the indications and technique of our current extra-articular augmentation procedure.

Extra-Articular Tenodesis in Combination with Anterior Cruciate Ligament Reconstruction: An Overview 87

Simone Cerciello, Cécile Batailler, Nader Darwich, and Philippe Neyret

Anterior cruciate ligament (ACL) reconstruction is a successful procedure with high rates of return to sport. However, some patients experience persistent instability and graft failure. These adverse events have a significant impact, especially on high-level athletes. In an effort to improve outcomes for these patients, more attention is being paid to the anatomic structures at the anterolateral aspect of the knee. The anterolateral structures of the knee have been shown to play a major role in decreasing rotatory knee instability and forces across the ACL graft following reconstruction. This article discusses the indications and techniques for anterolateral ligament reconstruction or lateral extra-articular tenodesis, along with the newest anatomic and biomechanics concepts.

The Role of an Extra-Articular Tenodesis in Revision of Anterior Cruciate Ligament Reconstruction 101

Thomas K. Miller

Patients who present for anterior cruciate ligament (ACL) revision with a high-grade pivot shift at the time of an index ACL revision procedure and subsequent reconstruction failure or a high-grade pivot shift at revision surgery, patients with generalized joint laxity, and those requiring soft tissue grafts should be considered candidates for lateral tenodesis to supplement intra-articular graft revision. Although there is no consensus regarding the optimal lateral tenodesis technique, due to the tibial positioning associated with tensioning and fixation of extra-articular procedures, a lateral tenodesis should not be used in patients with posterolateral corner injuries or lateral compartment articular disease.

Extra-Articular Plasty for Revision Anterior Cruciate Ligament Reconstruction   **115**

Panagiotis Ntagiopoulos and David Dejour

> Recent studies have renewed interest in the structures of the anterolateral aspect of the knee. Concomitant damage to these structures in the setting of anterior cruciate ligament rupture has led to various surgical techniques to address these combined injuries. This article is a description of the rationale and the indications for lateral extra-articular tenodesis as well as surgical technique.

The Influence of Tibial and Femoral Bone Morphology on Knee Kinematics in the Anterior Cruciate Ligament Injured Knee   **127**

Drew Lansdown and Chunbong Benjamin Ma

> Bone morphology is one feature that contributes to knee kinematics. The geometry of the tibia and femur vary across individuals, and these differences can influence the risk of anterior cruciate ligament (ACL) injury and of failure after isolated ACL reconstruction. There has been renewed interest in lateral extra-articular stabilization procedures to supplement an ACL reconstruction, although which patients benefit most from these procedures remains unclear. This article reviews the impact of bone morphology on knee kinematics, including tibial slope, depth of the medial tibial plateau, intercondylar notch shape, tibial eminence volume, and sphericity of the femoral condyles.

What Is the State of the Evidence in Anterolateral Ligament Research?   **137**

Paul A. Moroz, Emily E. Quick, Nolan S. Horner, Andrew Duong, Nicole Simunovic, and Olufemi R. Ayeni

> The anterolateral ligament (ALL) is a capsular structure of the knee that is the subject of increasing academic interest. This article reviewed recent ALL literature in terms of subject matter and quality. Although current literature focusing on the ALL is small and limited to level 4 and 5 evidence, it is rapidly expanding. Cadaveric studies describing ALL biomechanics are the most common study design, followed by radiographic studies. The methodologic quality of cadaveric studies focusing on the ALL is high. Clinically oriented research pertaining to the diagnosis, therapy, prevalence, or prognosis of injury to the ALL is presently lacking.

CLINICS IN SPORTS MEDICINE

FORTHCOMING ISSUES

April 2018
Common Procedures, Common Problems
Mark D. Miller, *Editor*

July 2018
Statistics in Sports Medicine
Stephen Thompson and Joe Hart, *Editors*

October 2018
Shoulder Arthritis in the Young and Active Patient
Stephen F. Brockmeier and
Brian C. Werner, *Editors*

RECENT ISSUES

October 2017
The Female Athlete
Siobhan M. Statuta, *Editor*

July 2017
Articular Cartilage
Eric C. McCarty, *Editor*

April 2017
Facial Injuries in Sports
Michael J. Stuart, *Editor*

RELATED INTEREST

Physical Medicine and Rehabilitation Clinics of North America, February 2016
(Vol. 27, Issue 1)
Running Injuries
Adam S. Tenforde, *Editor*
Available at: http://www.pmr.theclinics.com/

THE CLINICS ARE AVAILABLE ONLINE!
Access your subscription at:
www.theclinics.com

Erratum

In the article "Exercise in Pregnancy" by Vanessa H. Gregg, MD, in the October issue of *Clinics in Sports Medicine* (Volume 36, Issue 4) the following sources should have appeared:

For Box 1, "Relative Contraindications to Aerobic Exercise During Pregnancy": Reprinted with permission from Physical activity and exercise during pregnancy and the postpartum period. Committee Opinion No.650. American College of Obstetricians and Gynecologists. Obstet Gynecol 2015 :126:e135-42.

For Box 2, "Absolute Contraindications to Aerobic Exercise During Pregnancy": Reprinted with permission from Physical activity and exercise during pregnancy and the postpartum period. Committee Opinion No.650. American College of Obstetricians and Gynecologists. Obstet Gynecol 2015 :126:e135-42.

For Box 3, "Warning Signs to Discontinue Exercise While Pregnant": Reprinted with permission from Physical activity and exercise during pregnancy and the postpartum period. Committee Opinion No.650. American College of Obstetricians and Gynecologists. Obstet Gynecol 2015 :126:e135-42.

For Table 3, "Risks of Exercise in Pregnancy for the Elite Athlete": Reprinted with permission from Artal R, Hopkins S. Exercise. Clin Update Womens Health Care 2013;XII(2):1-105.

Clin Sports Med 37 (2018) xiii
https://doi.org/10.1016/j.csm.2017.10.003
0278-5919/18/© 2017 Elsevier Inc. All rights reserved.

Foreword

ALL or None?

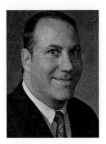

Mark D. Miller, MD
Consulting Editor

The debate regarding the existence, function, location, and reconstruction of the ante-rolateral ligament (ALL) of the knee continues. Because of his tremendous experience in anterior cruciate ligament (ACL) reconstruction, and his active role in this debate, I invited my mentor, Dr Freddie Fu, to put together a treatise on this subject. He invited an international consortium of ACL experts to make their case. He has covered all aspects without any bias, leaving it up to you, the reader, to make the call. I personally believe that there is some importance to anterolateral structures in ACL instability, regardless of what you call it, but, like many of you, I have not fully committed to performing ALL reconstruction in most patients. There may be a role in complex revision procedures with significant rotatory instability, but it remains unclear whether an ALL reconstruction with a free graft or a tenodesis of a portion of the iliotibial band is the best option. There is much study currently underway, and we should all carefully follow this research and continue to ask questions as we continue to seek the best for our patients.

Mark D. Miller, MD
S. Ward Casscells Professor
Division of Sports Medicine
Department of Orthopaedic Surgery
University of Virginia
400 Ray C. Hunt Drive, Suite 330
Charlottesville, VA 22908-0159, USA

E-mail address:
mdm3p@virginia.edu

Clin Sports Med 37 (2018) xv
https://doi.org/10.1016/j.csm.2017.10.002
0278-5919/18/© 2017 Published by Elsevier Inc.

sportsmed.theclinics.com

Preface

Structures of the Anterolateral Knee: Why All the Confusion?

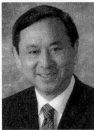 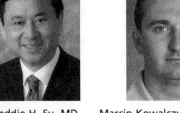

Freddie H. Fu, MD   Marcin Kowalczuk, MD, FRCSC
                       Editors

Over the last two decades we have seen a shift in anterior cruciate ligament (ACL) reconstruction that focuses on restoration of the native anatomy. Despite this anatomic approach, a subset of patients continue to experience anterolateral rotatory instability. This persistent instability suggests that pieces to the puzzle that is complex knee instability are still missing. Continued efforts to improve clinical outcomes have led to the recent resurgence of interest in the anatomic structures of the anterolateral knee, termed the anterolateral complex (ALC). Most notably this has yielded a significant body of literature regarding the anterolateral ligament (ALL). This renewed interest has led to healthy academic debate as well as significant confusion.

The confusion stems from the inherent complexity of the lateral knee anatomy. Historically the structures of the ALC and ALL have gone by many names, which has contributed to inconsistencies of anatomic nomenclature.[1] Many of these inconsistencies are due to differences in dissection technique and the variable use of embalmed versus fresh frozen specimens in study protocols. The process of tissue embalming changes tissue consistency and blurs important planes of dissection. This is of paramount importance when discerning the difference between capsular thickenings and discrete ligamentous tissues. The aforementioned factors have all contributed to the confusion regarding the anatomic structures of the ALC and ALL. A lack of consensus on anatomic nomenclature naturally translates into a poor understanding of function, which can be seen in the variable results across biomechanical studies of the ALC and ALL.

In an effort to correct or prevent residual anterolateral knee instability, orthopedic surgeons have increasingly turned to lateral tenodesis and reconstruction procedures. These lateral procedures, while potentially decreasing rotatory instability, can also lead to overconstraint, increased external tibial rotation, and greater contact stresses in the lateral compartment.[2,3] Although the body of literature regarding the ALC and ALL

Clin Sports Med 37 (2018) xvii–xviii
https://doi.org/10.1016/j.csm.2017.10.001
0278-5919/18/© 2017 Published by Elsevier Inc.

continues to grow, it is chiefly limited to cadaveric studies and case series. High-level studies in the form of randomized clinical trials are on the horizon, but for the time being augmentation of ACL reconstruction with lateral procedures should be approached with caution and considered in each patient individually. Surgical indications remain unclear, and undue long-term harm remains a distinct possibility.

The puzzle that is complex knee instability continues to challenge clinicians. It is important to remember that the pivot shift phenomenon is multifactorial, with bone morphology, ligamentous laxity, meniscal tissues, and the posterolateral and anterolateral structures all playing contributory roles.[4] The anterolateral knee structures are a critical piece of the puzzle but have also been the source of considerable confusion. In an effort to provide clarity, we hope that this special issue of *Clinics in Sports Medicine* authored by an international panel of experts will provide an open arena for the exchange of knowledge and critical appraisal of the literature. With an improved understanding of anatomy, biomechanic function, and surgical indications, improved patient outcomes in this challenging patient population can be achieved.

Freddie H. Fu, MD
Department of Orthopaedic Surgery
University of Pittsburgh
UPMC Center for Sports Medicine
3200 South Water Street
Pittsburgh, PA 15203, USA

Marcin Kowalczuk, MD, FRCSC
Department of Orthopaedic Surgery
University of Pittsburgh
UPMC Center for Sports Medicine
3200 South Water Street
Pittsburgh, PA 15203, USA

E-mail addresses:
ffu@upmc.edu (F.H. Fu)
kowalczukm@upmc.edu (M. Kowalczuk)

REFERENCES

1. Cavaignac E, Ancelin D, Chiron P, et al. Historical perspective on the "discovery" of the anterolateral ligament of the knee. Knee Surg Sports Traumatol Arthrosc 2017;25(4):991–6.
2. Inderhaug E, Stephen JM, Williams A, et al. Biomechanical comparison of anterolateral procedures combined with anterior cruciate ligament reconstruction. Am J Sports Med 2017;45(2):347–54.
3. Slette EL, Mikula JD, Schon JM, et al. Biomechanical results of lateral extra-articular tenodesis procedures of the knee: a systematic review. Arthroscopy 2016; 32(12):2592–611.
4. Fu FH, Herbst E. Editorial commentary: the pivot-shift phenomenon is multifactorial. Arthroscopy 2016;32(6):1063–4.

A Layered Anatomic Description of the Anterolateral Complex of the Knee

Marcin Kowalczuk, MD, FRCSC[a], Elmar Herbst, MD[a,b],
Jeremy M. Burnham, MD[a], Marcio Albers, MD[a],
Volker Musahl, MD[a], Freddie H. Fu, MD[a,*]

KEYWORDS

• Anterolateral complex • Knee • Iliotibial band • Capsule • Anterolateral ligament

KEY POINTS

• Variability in anatomic terminology, dissection protocols, and the use of embalmed as opposed to fresh frozen specimens has led to the controversy surrounding the anterolateral structures of the knee.

• The complex anatomy of the anterolateral knee is made up of the many layers of the iliotibial band, the underlying capsule, and its direct attachments to the lateral meniscus.

• The iliotibial band is composed of the superficial, middle, deep, and capsulo-osseous layers.

• Collectively these structures are termed the anterolateral complex of the knee.

• The anterolateral complex of the knee works synergistically with adjacent meniscal tissue and meniscal roots to resist internal tibial rotation.

INTRODUCTION

The goal of improving rotatory knee stability in patients undergoing anterior cruciate ligament (ACL) reconstruction has led to renewed interest in the extra-articular structures of the anterolateral knee and description of the proposed anterolateral ligament (ALL).[1–4] Although the principal function of the anterolateral knee structures in resisting internal tibial rotation is generally accepted, the exact itemized anatomic structures and their respective contributions to resisting internal tibial rotation remain unclear.[5]

Disclosure Statement: The authors collectively declare they have no conflicts of interest.
[a] Department of Orthopaedic Surgery, University of Pittsburgh, UPMC Center for Sports Medicine, 3200 South Water Street, Pittsburgh, PA 15203, USA; [b] Department of Orthopaedic Sports Medicine, Klinikum rechts der Isar, Technical University Munich, Ismaninger Street 22, 81675 Munich, Germany
* Corresponding author.
E-mail address: ffu@upmc.edu

Clin Sports Med 37 (2018) 1–8
http://dx.doi.org/10.1016/j.csm.2017.07.001
0278-5919/18/© 2017 Elsevier Inc. All rights reserved.

sportsmed.theclinics.com

In examining the ever-expanding body of literature on the topic, differences in anatomic terminology have resulted in inconsistency in the orthopedic literature. Although some experts describe a distinct ligamentous structure at the anterolateral aspect of the knee, other scientific reports show that the observed resistance to internal tibial rotation is secondary to a multitude of anterolateral tissues working synergistically.[6] This confluence of tissues or anterolateral complex (ALC) of the knee is described in this review.[7]

THE LAYERS OF THE LATERAL ASPECT OF THE KNEE

The lateral structures of the knee conceptually are often grouped into enveloping layers. Seebacher and colleagues[8] grouped the anatomic structures of the lateral knee into 3 layers, analogous to Warren and Marshall's description of the medial structures of the knee.[9] In contrast to the medial side, the layered individual structures of the lateral side are more complex and at times difficult to discern.

Layer I consists of the iliotibial band (ITB) and its anterior and posterior expansions.[8] Layer II anteriorly is represented by the retinaculum of the quadriceps (patellar retinaculum). Posteriorly, layer II is incomplete and is represented by attachments to the lateral intermuscular septum, posterolateral capsule, and lateral head of the gastrocnemius. Layer III is chiefly composed of the tibiofemoral joint capsule, which posterior to the ITB divides into a superficial and deep layer. Housed between the superficial and deep capsular layers is the lateral collateral ligament (LCL), and medial to it, the inferior lateral geniculate artery.[8] The superficial capsular layer terminates posteriorly when it meets the fabellofibular ligament, and the deep layer forms the coronary ligaments to the lateral meniscus and then blends with the arcuate ligament further posteriorly.[8,10]

THE ANTEROLATERAL COMPLEX

Anterolaterally from superficial to deep the knee is enveloped by the ITB with its associated deeper layers, and the joint capsule. Collectively, these structures are termed the ALC.[7] The dominant structure encountered is the ITB and although appearing as a simple thick band of tissue attaching to the Gerdy tubercle, the ITB is in fact complex and composed of a multitude of layers.

THE SUPERFICIAL AND MIDDLE LAYERS OF THE ILIOTIBIAL BAND

The superficial layer of the ITB proximally is firmly adhered to the linea aspera via connections to the lateral intermuscular septum.[4] Distally, the anterior aspect of the superficial layer is identified by its characteristic curved fibers attaching to the lateral patella and patellar tendon.[11] These "arciform fibers," which blend with the fascia of the patella, were first described by Kaplan[12] and run at 70° to 80° compared with fibers heading toward the Gerdy tubercle.[4] In the literature, the anterior fibers of the superficial layer of the ITB have also been termed the "iliopatellar band" or "superficial oblique retinaculum."[13,14] The central fibers of the superficial layer distally insert in a fanlike fashion on and around the Gerdy tubercle[4] (**Fig. 1**). Further posteriorly, the superficial layer terminates as a fascia that reinforces the biceps femoris.[8,14]

Immediately deep and directly adherent to the superficial layer is the middle layer of the ITB, which can be identified only with careful sharp dissection and serves to reinforce the structural integrity of the superficial layer.[14] The middle layer can be identified by its characteristic fibers, which run from lateral proximal to medial distal, which is in contrast to the vertical nature of the superficial ITB fibers.[14]

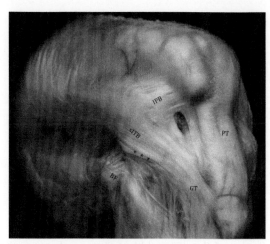

Fig. 1. The superficial iliotibial band (sITB) and posterior to this, the fascia of the biceps femoris (BF) muscle are depicted. Anterior to the sITB the iliopatellar band (IPB) inserts on the lateral patella and patellar tendon (PT). At 90° of knee flexion, the posterior part of the sITB becomes folded. GT, Gerdy tubercle. (*From* Herbst E, Albers M, Burnham JM, et al. The anterolateral complex of the knee: a pictorial essay. Knee Surg Sports Traumatol Arthrosc 2017;25(4):1010; with permission.)

THE DEEP LAYER OF THE ILIOTIBIAL BAND

The deep layer of the ITB lies posterior and medial to the superficial and middle layers. Its origin is at the lateral femoral supracondylar area and stretches approximately 6 cm proximally, just distal to the end of the lateral intermuscular septum.[14] Reflection of the superficial layer will reveal the deep layer of the ITB fanning out in the coronal plane and curving distally before becoming confluent with the aforementioned superficial and middle layers distally.

Close examination of the fibers, which make up the origin of deep layer of the ITB from distal to proximal, reveals discrete thickening in the supracondylar region. These deep fibers just distal to the intermuscular septum and in close proximity to the traversing superior geniculate vessels are termed the Kaplan fibers.[15] This deep femorotibial connection of the ITB was also described by Lobenhoffer and colleagues,[16] as they noted a distinct set of transverse running ITB fibers just distal to the intermuscular septum that were followed even farther distally by "retrograde fiber tracts," which traversed from the Gerdy tubercle back to the femur in a more arcuate fashion.

THE CAPSULO-OSSEOUS LAYER OF THE ILIOTIBIAL BAND

The capsulo-osseous layer of the ITB is considered a distinct layer by some, whereas other studies report it to be an indistinguishable component of the deep layer[4,6,10,14,16] (**Fig. 2**). Nonetheless, given its unique structure and proposed function, it deserves specific mention. The capsulo-osseous layer of the ITB is located more posteriorly compared with those that run superficial to it. At its posterior margin, the capsulo-osseous layer is continuous with the fascia of the gastrocnemius and plantaris muscles.[14] Posteriorly, there is also an attachment of the short of biceps femoris, which Terry and LaPrade[17] termed the biceps-capsulo-osseous iliotibial tract confluens. Distally, the capsulo-osseous layer inserts posterior to and distal to the Gerdy

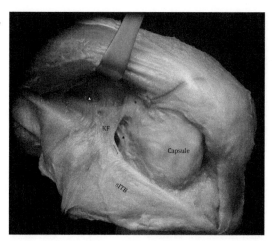

Fig. 2. Posterior reflection of the sITB and blunt dissection between the deep ITB (*black arrow*) and the anterolateral capsule reveals the capsulo-osseous layer (*black arrowhead*). In close proximity to branches of the superior genicular artery (*white arrowhead*), the Kaplan fibers (KF) can be seen originating from the distal femoral metaphysis and lateral supraepicondylar region (*asterisk* shows the accessory fiber bundles of the KF). (*From* Herbst E, Albers M, Burnham JM, et al. The anterolateral complex of the knee: a pictorial essay. Knee Surg Sports Traumatol Arthrosc 2017;25(4):1011; with permission.)

tubercle, and proximally its origin is located on the lateral supraepicondylar region bordering the lateral epicondyle.[4] As it runs to its aforementioned insertion, the capsulo-osseous layer lies immediately superficial to the anterolateral capsule of the knee joint.

THE ANTEROLATERAL CAPSULE

The lateral capsulo-ligamentous architecture has been described by Hughston and colleagues[18] and is divided into the anterior, middle, and posterior thirds. The structures of the anterior third include the capsule and overlying quadriceps retinaculum, stretching from the lateral border of the patella and patellar tendon to the anterior border of the superficial ITB. The superficial ITB and the layers deep to it, including the joint capsule, form the middle third capsular layer, which extends posteriorly to the anterior border of the LCL. The joint capsule of the knee naturally thickens to stabilize the lateral meniscus in the form of the meniscotibial and meniscofemoral ligaments[19,20] (**Fig. 3**). This middle third layer is anchored proximally at the femoral epicondyle and distally at the tibial joint line. The posterior third structures, which include the LCL, arcuate ligament, popliteus, and underlying joint capsule, are collectively termed the arcuate complex.[18]

THE "ANTEROLATERAL LIGAMENT"

The anatomic description of the ALL has varied in the literature. Claes and colleagues[1] described the ALL as a discrete ligament with attachments to the lateral meniscus, originating from the lateral femoral epicondyle and inserting just distal to the tibial joint line between the fibular head and Gerdy tubercle. In contrast, the ALL also has been described as a distinctly extracapsular structure originating 8.0 mm proximal and 4.3 mm posterior to the lateral epicondyle coursing superficial to the LCL with no direct

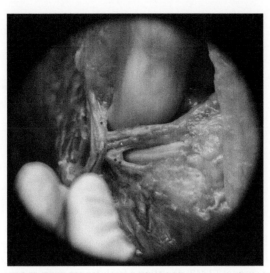

Fig. 3. A thickening of the lateral knee capsule forms the coronary ligament, which is made up of the meniscofemoral (*asterisks*) and meniscotibial (*double asterisks*) ligaments. Medial to the coronary ligament, the inferior genicular artery (*white arrowhead*) runs anteriorly. (*From* Herbst E, Albers M, Burnham JM, et al. The anterolateral complex of the knee: a pictorial essay. Knee Surg Sports Traumatol Arthrosc 2017;25(4):1012; with permission.)

attachments to the lateral meniscal rim.[21] This is contrary to alternate descriptions of the ALL as a thickening of the anterolateral capsule with an origin that is anterior and distal to the femoral epicondyle.[22] In a recent MRI study on human cadaveric specimens, such a thickening of the anterolateral capsule was identified in only 3 of 10 specimens. As measured on 3T MRI, the thickness of the anterolateral capsule at its greatest dimension never exceeded 3.3 mm[23] (**Fig. 4**). The overall prevalence of a capsular thickening or "ALL" has been reported to be from 12.5% to 100% in fresh frozen cadaver knee specimens in the recent literature.[3,23–26]

When comparing the proposed locations of the ALL with classic literature, it may be possible that investigators are referring to either the capsulo-osseous layer of the ITB or the mid-third capsular ligament, as described by Hughston and colleagues.[18] Terry and colleagues[14,17] described the capsulo-osseous layer of the ITB, which "acts as an anterolateral ligament of the knee," particularly as the knee approaches extension. This capsulo-osseous layer along with portions of the deep layer is what is likely the ligamentum femoro-tibiale laterale anterius described by Müller,[27] the "retrograde fiber tracts" of Lobenhoffer and colleagues[16] or what Hassler and Jakob[28] described as the ligamentum tractotibiale. The anatomic descriptions of these fiber tracts of the ITB (from lateral supraepicondylar to an area posterior to the Gerdy tubercle) would be in line with some of recent descriptions of the ALL.[21,29] However, none of the recent studies described the proximal continuity of these fiber tracts with the fascia of the lateral gastrocnemius and plantaris muscles.[14]

When compared with the deep and capsulo-osseus layer of the ITB, the anterolateral capsule provides little restraint to internal tibial rotation.[6,30] Biomechanical data have shown that the anterolateral capsule does not effectively transmit forces longitudinally between the tibia and femur like a ligament, but rather functions as sheet of fibrous tissue and aids in dissipating forces to neighboring structures.[31] During robotic pivot shift testing using human cadaveric specimens, the anterolateral capsule experiences

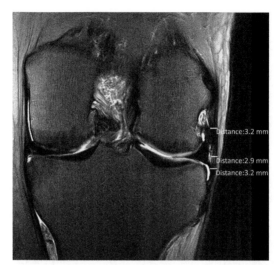

Distance:3.2 mm
Distance:2.9 mm
Distance:3.2 mm

Fig. 4. Predissection coronal T2 MRI depicting a fresh-frozen cadaveric specimen with thickening of the lateral capsule and accompanying measurements. Measurements documented the thickness (in a medial–lateral plane) of the thickening proximally (measured at the caudal margin of the sulcus for the popliteus insertion), in the midportion (measured at the mid-meniscus level) and distally (measured at the level of the subchondral plate of the lateral tibial plateau). On this specimen, measurements equaled: proximal, 3.2 mm; midportion, 2.9 mm; and distal, 3.2 mm. (*From* Dombrowski ME, Costello JM, Ohashi B, et al. Macroscopic anatomic, histologic and magnetic resonance imaging correlation of the lateral capsule of the knee. Knee Surg Sports Traumatol Arthrosc 2016;24(9):2856; with permission.)

relatively low in situ forces compared with the ACL and overlying anterolateral tissues.[30] Although a thickening of the capsule anterolaterally can be appreciated in 30% to 40% of cases, biomechanical studies have shown its stiffness and ultimate load is much lower than comparable capsular tissue from the posteromedial aspect of the knee.[5] This is contrary to what would be expected if ligamentous tissues were present. This suggests that the capsule instead works synergistically with the layers of the ALC, adjacent meniscal tissue, and meniscal roots to control rotatory knee instability.[5,32,33]

SUMMARY

The anatomy of the ALC is multifaceted and conceptually can be divided into the superficial, middle, deep, and capsulo-osseous layers of the ITB, which overlie the anterolateral joint capsule, including the mid-third capsular ligament. Collectively, these structures form the ALC of the knee, which in conjunction with the ACL is believed to be important in preventing anterolateral rotatory instability. Future large-scale clinical studies will be necessary to better understand the multiple factors that influence anterolateral rotatory knee instability. As our knowledge of the anterolateral structures of the knee develops, the goal continues to be improved diagnosis and treatment of complex knee injuries. Ultimately, the goal will be improved outcomes for patients with rotatory instability secondary to ACL injury.

REFERENCES

1. Claes S, Vereecke E, Maes M, et al. Anatomy of the anterolateral ligament of the knee. J Anat 2013;223(4):321–8.

2. Kennedy MI, Claes S, Fuso FA, et al. The anterolateral ligament: an anatomic, radiographic, and biomechanical analysis. Am J Sports Med 2015;43(7): 1606–15.

3. Van der Watt L, Khan M, Rothrauff BB, et al. The structure and function of the anterolateral ligament of the knee: a systematic review. Arthroscopy 2015;31(3): 569–82.e3.

4. Vieira EL, Vieira EA, da Silva RT, et al. An anatomic study of the iliotibial tract. Arthroscopy 2007;23(3):269–74.

5. Rahnemai-Azar AA, Miller RM, Guenther D, et al. Structural properties of the anterolateral capsule and iliotibial band of the knee. Am J Sports Med 2016;44(4): 892–7.

6. Kittl C, El-Daou H, Athwal KK, et al. The role of the anterolateral structures and the ACL in controlling laxity of the intact and ACL-deficient knee. Am J Sports Med 2016;44(2):345–54.

7. Herbst E, Albers M, Burnham JM, et al. The anterolateral complex of the knee: a pictorial essay. Knee Surg Sports Traumatol Arthrosc 2017;25(4):1009–14.

8. Seebacher JR, Inglis AE, Marshall JL, et al. The structure of the posterolateral aspect of the knee. J Bone Joint Surg Am 1982;64(4):536–41.

9. Warren LF, Marshall JL. The supporting structures and layers on the medial side of the knee: an anatomical analysis. J Bone Joint Surg Am 1979;61(1):56–62.

10. Kaplan EB. Some aspects of functional anatomy of the human knee joint. Clin Orthop 1962;23:18–29.

11. Merican AM, Amis AA. Anatomy of the lateral retinaculum of the knee. J Bone Joint Surg Br 2008;90(4):527–34.

12. Kaplan EB. Surgical approach to the lateral (peroneal) side of the knee joint. Surg Gynecol Obstet 1957;104(3):346–56.

13. Fulkerson JP, Gossling HR. Anatomy of the knee joint lateral retinaculum. Clin Orthop Relat Res 1980;153:183–8.

14. Terry GC, Hughston JC, Norwood LA. The anatomy of the iliopatellar band and iliotibial tract. Am J Sports Med 1986;14(1):39–45.

15. Kaplan EB. The iliotibial tract; clinical and morphological significance. J Bone Joint Surg Am 1958;40A(4):817–32.

16. Lobenhoffer P, Posel P, Witt S, et al. Distal femoral fixation of the iliotibial tract. Arch Orthop Trauma Surg 1987;106(5):285–90.

17. Terry GC, LaPrade RF. The biceps femoris muscle complex at the knee. Its anatomy and injury patterns associated with acute anterolateral-anteromedial rotatory instability. Am J Sports Med 1996;24(1):2–8.

18. Hughston JC, Andrews JR, Cross MJ, et al. Classification of knee ligament instabilities. Part II. The lateral compartment. J Bone Joint Surg Am 1976;58(2):173–9.

19. Hughston JC, Andrews JR, Cross MJ, et al. Classification of knee ligament instabilities. Part I. The medial compartment and cruciate ligaments. J Bone Joint Surg Am 1976;58(2):159–72.

20. Corbo G, Norris M, Getgood A, et al. The infra-meniscal fibers of the anterolateral ligament are stronger and stiffer than the supra-meniscal fibers despite similar histological characteristics. Knee Surg Sports Traumatol Arthrosc 2017;25(4): 1078–85.

21. Dodds AL, Halewood C, Gupte CM, et al. The anterolateral ligament: anatomy, length changes and association with the Segond fracture. Bone Joint J 2014; 96B(3):325–31.

22. Caterine S, Litchfield R, Johnson M, et al. A cadaveric study of the anterolateral ligament: re-introducing the lateral capsular ligament. Knee Surg Sports Traumatol Arthrosc 2015;23(11):3186–95.
23. Dombrowski ME, Costello JM, Ohashi B, et al. Macroscopic anatomical, histological and magnetic resonance imaging correlation of the lateral capsule of the knee. Knee Surg Sports Traumatol Arthrosc 2016;24(9):2854–60.
24. Roessler PP, Schuttler KF, Stein T, et al. Anatomic dissection of the anterolateral ligament (ALL) in paired fresh-frozen cadaveric knee joints. Arch Orthop Trauma Surg 2017;137(2):249–55.
25. Shea KG, Milewski MD, Cannamela PC, et al. Anterolateral ligament of the knee shows variable anatomy in pediatric specimens. Clin Orthop Relat Res 2016; 475(6):1583–91.
26. Shea KG, Polousky JD, Jacobs JC Jr, et al. The anterolateral ligament of the knee: an inconsistent finding in pediatric cadaveric specimens. J Pediatr Orthop 2016; 36(5):e51–4.
27. Müller W. Das Knie. Form, Funktion und ligamentaere Wiederherstellungschirurgie. Berlin/Heidelberg/New York: Springer; 1982.
28. Hassler H, Jakob RP. On the cause of the anterolateral instability of the knee joint. A study on 20 cadaver knee joints with special regard to the tractus iliotibialis (author's transl). Arch Orthop Trauma Surg 1981;98(1):45–50 [in German].
29. Daggett M, Busch K, Sonnery-Cottet B. Surgical dissection of the anterolateral ligament. Arthrosc Tech 2016;5(1):e185–8.
30. Bell KM, Rahnemai-Azar AA, Irarrazaval S, et al. In-situ forces in the anterolateral capsule resulting from a simulated pivot shift test. Orthopaedic Research Society Annual Meeting. Lake Buena Vista (FL), March 5, 2016.
31. Guenther D, Rahnemai-Azar AA, Bell KM, et al. The anterolateral capsule of the knee behaves like a sheet of fibrous tissue. Am J Sports Med 2016;45(4):849–55.
32. Musahl V, Citak M, O'Loughlin PF, et al. The effect of medial versus lateral meniscectomy on the stability of the anterior cruciate ligament-deficient knee. Am J Sports Med 2010;38(8):1591–7.
33. Shybut TB, Vega CE, Haddad J, et al. Effect of lateral meniscal root tear on the stability of the anterior cruciate ligament-deficient knee. Am J Sports Med 2015;43(4):905–11.

The Anterolateral Ligament Does Exist

An Anatomic Description

Stefano Zaffagnini, MD[a,b], Alberto Grassi, MD[a,b],
Giulio Maria Marcheggiani Muccioli, MD[a,b],
Federico Raggi, MD[a,b], Matteo Romagnoli, MD[c], Alice Bondi, MD[c],
Salvatore Calderone, MD[c], Cecilia Signorelli, PhD[b,*]

KEYWORDS

- Anterior cruciate ligament • Anterolateral ligament • ACL • ALL
- Anterolateral capsule • Knee anatomy

KEY POINTS

- The existence, precise anatomy, and role of the anterolateral ligament (ALL) represent the principal sources of recent controversy among orthopedic surgeons.
- The present article investigates the historical, phylogenetic, anatomic, arthroscopic and radiological evidence regarding the ALL.
- Caused by/because of the confusing terminology, different dissection technique and specimen's characteristics, an agreement still cannot be reached among the experts regarding the ALL existence, anatomy and function.

INTRODUCTION

The debate around the existence, anatomy, and role of the so-called anterolateral ligament" (ALL) represents one of the principal sources of controversy among the orthopedic community. Since the landmark study by Claes and colleagues,[1] in 2013, which renewed interest in the anterolateral anatomy of the knee, many efforts have been made to try to reconcile historical theories with modern anatomic and biomechanical findings. The burden of this topic is made evident by the more than 130 studies

Disclosure: The authors declare no relationship with commercial companies that has a direct financial interest in subject matter or materials discussed in this article or with a company making a competing product.
[a] 2nd Orthopaedic and Traumatologic Clinic, Istituto Ortopedico Rizzoli, Via Di Barbiano 1/10, Bologna 40136, Italy; [b] Laboratory of Biomechanics and Technology Innovation, Istituto Ortopedico Rizzoli, Via Di Barbiano 1/10, Bologna 40136, Italy; [c] Rizzoli-Sicilia Department, Istituto Ortopedico Rizzoli, SS (State motorway) 113, km 246, Bagheria 90011, Palermo, Italy
* Corresponding author.
E-mail address: c.signorelli@biomec.ior.it

available on PubMed at the time of the current article's preparation, under the term "knee anterolateral ligament."

Despite these extensive research efforts, there is still no consensus on whether or not the ALL exists and which functions it serves. A consensus meeting among the ALL experts took place in Lyon, France, in November 2015 to exchange clinical and research experiences in order to clarify the main aspects related to the topic of the ALL, which have been summarized in a consensus paper.[2] The investigators concluded that "the ALL is a distinct ligament of the anterolateral side of the human knee."[2] However, other investigators still refute this statement, denying the presence of a true ligament and citing the importance of other anatomic structures such as the anterolateral capsule and the deep portion of the iliotibial band (ITB).[3–5] Whether this disagreement is matter of terminology or dissection techniques has yet to be determined. Nevertheless, given the large volume of evidence, the presence of an anatomic structure at the anterolateral aspect of the knee, with an oblique course from the lateral epicondyle to the proximal tibia, should be acknowledged. This structure, which tightens in internal rotation, has been repeatedly described and investigated by several investigators over the last 2 centuries.[6–13]

This article presents and discusses the historical and anatomic evidence that supports the presence of a real and well-defined ALL.

HISTORICAL PROOF

Despite the development of the modern concept of ALL being universally considered to have occurred, with much media attention, in October 2013 after the report of Claes and colleagues,[1] the term ALL had already been used 1 year earlier by Vincent and colleagues[14,15] to describe a ligamentous structure of the anterolateral part of the knee isolated during total knee arthroplasty. Despite this, Claes and colleagues[1] claimed to be the first to systematically describe, in both a qualitative and quantitative manner, a "well defined ligamentous structure, clearly distinguishable from the anterolateral joint capsule"[1] with an "origin situated at the prominence of lateral femoral epicondyle, [...] an oblique course [...], firm attachments to the lateral meniscus"[1] and an "insertion on the anterolateral tibia [...] grossly located midway between Gerdy's tubercle and the tip of fibular head, definitely separated from the iliotibial band."[1] Despite this breakthrough, the first reports of the structure date back more than a century.

The main and, at times, inappropriately cited reference of the ALL is the 1879 study by the French Gynecologist Paul Ferdinand Segond.[10] Segond[10] described an intra-articular crack, fissure, or bone wound of the anterolateral portion of the tibia's lateral condylar surface during autopsy observations of knees that were forcefully rotated. He also described a "pearly, resistant, fibrous band that is placed under extreme tension when the knee is forcefully internally rotated",[10] which is now advocated to be the ALL. An accurate description of the structure's origin, insertion, or dimensions along with dissection technique was not provided. Similarly, the German anatomist Josias Weitbrecht[13] in 1752, more than a century before Segond, described "fibrous bunches that reinforce the capsule and bands that supplement the fixation of semicircular cartilage (meniscus)."[13] However, as in the case of Segond,[10] no precise description was provided.

Cavaignac and colleagues,[16] in a recent historical essay on the ALL, reported that several works from the late 1800s and early 1900s, consistently described a "lateral epicondilo-meniscal ligament." The German Anatomist Friedrich Henle, in 1871, noted that "the most anterior fibers of the lateral collateral ligament curve forward at nearly right angle and disappear into the edge of the meniscus."[6] Several years later, around 1920, French anatomists Vallois[12] and Jost[8] confirmed and expanded on this anatomic description by reporting a structure "arising from the lateral femoral epicondyle [...]. Through an oblique anteroinferior course, and after getting slightly wider, it attaches to the superior and peripheral edge of anterior horn of the lateral meniscus [...]. It ends at the tibia."[8,12]

Moving to the modern era of sports medicine, several authoritative surgeons gave their contributions to the understanding of the anatomy of the lateral aspect of the knee. In the 1970s, Hughston and colleagues[7] (Jack Hughston is known as the father of American sports medicine), described the "the middle third of the lateral capsular ligament"[7] as "technically strong"[7] and as a "major lateral static support around 30° of flexion."[7] A few years later, Werner Müller in Europe described a structure extending from the linea aspera of the femur to the Gerdy tubercle.[9] Anatomic studies by Terry and colleagues[11] in 1993 described an interconnection between anterior cruciate ligament (ACL) and the "capsulo-osseous layer of ITB"; the latter, running from the epicondylar region to the proximal tibia. It was suggested that these distinct fibers of the ITB create with the ACL an inverse U (horseshoe) structure around the posterior aspect of the lateral femoral condyle.

On review of previously published literature, the structure that is currently referred to as the ALL has been the subject of numerous but discordant studies. However, because of a lack of accurate anatomic descriptions and inconsistent terminology, it is impossible to link these historical descriptions to the modern ALL concept without some degree of speculation.

PHYLOGENETIC PROOF

Evidence for the existence of an ALL also derives from its presence in an evolutionary context. Cavaignac and colleagues,[16] in their historical essay, highlighted the anthropologic studies of Vallois[12] and Jost.[8] The French anatomists, who described the presence of a lateral epicondilo-meniscal ligament in humans, also reported its presence in *Tarsius*, lemur, *Perodicticus*, and gibbons.[8,12] They also considered that the ligament was "particularly well developed in animals requiring control over rotational stability of their knee, particularly in climbers".[16] However, a recent anatomic study of various animal species, such as bonobo, gorilla, lemur, deer, gazelle, bear, kangaroo, and tiger, reported opposite results, citing no evidence of an ALL.[17]

The embryology of the ALL has been investigated in human fetal and pediatric specimens.[18–20] The Brazilian group of Helito and colleagues[18] performed a surgical dissection of 20 fetal embalmed knees aged 25.5 to 37.3 weeks with a mean length of 40 cm. After the fascia lata was dissected to its distal insertion, the ALL was isolated during knee flexion and internal rotation in all the specimens. The femoral insertion around the femoral epicondyle and the tibial insertion midway between the Gerdy and fibular head were consistent with data reported by Claes and colleagues.[1] However, the length and width were 6 times shorter and 4 times narrower than those of adult specimens. The same investigators, on histologic evaluation, found well-organized connective tissue similar to the ligamentous tissue found in adults but with increased cellularity. These observations are in contrast with the findings of Sabzevari and colleagues,[19] who did not report a distinct ligamentous structure to be present in a sample of 21 fresh fetal knees aged 18 to 22 weeks. The investigators, who identified all of the other knee ligamentous structures except for the ALL, theorized that capsular thickening develops in some individuals because of different loads applied to the knee capsule.[19] Shea and colleagues[20] similarly reported on the inconsistent presence of the ALL in pediatric specimens with a median age of 8 years. Several anatomic variations of the ALL were described in 64% of specimens. In conclusion, from an evolutionary and developmental point of view, the presence of the ALL seems to be supported. However, controversy remains and additional studies are needed.

ANATOMIC PROOF

The most significant debate with regard to the ALL surrounds its anatomy. According to the consensus paper from the ALL Expert Group, the ALL is considered a "distinct ligament at the anterolateral side of the human knee,"[2] "deep to the iliotibial band,"[2] with "femoral attachment [...] posterior and proximal to the lateral epicondyle, and a tibial attachment [...] between Gerdy's tubercle and the fibular head"[2] with a "constant attachment to the lateral meniscus."[2] These statements have been supported by many anatomic studies, which have reported the incidence of the ALL to be between 50% and 100% in cadaveric specimens drawn from several populations (Table 1).[21–30] According to Daggett and colleagues,[31] the ALL can be identified reflecting distally from the ITB up to its insertion at the Gerdy tubercle, after a transverse incision is made 6 to 8 cm proximal to the lateral epicondyle. Because the proximal ALL is reported to be closely adhered to the ITB, tissue must be carefully reflected at this point.[31] Applying internal rotation with the knee flexed between 30° and 60°, the oblique fanlike fibers of the ALL can be seen running from the epicondylar region to the proximal tibia and attaching between the Gerdy tubercle and the fibular head (Fig. 1). On reflecting the biceps femoris insertion on the fibula posteriorly, the lateral collateral ligament (LCL) can be seen and the capsule between the LCL and ALL can be excised by sharp dissection. By also excising the capsule anterior to the ALL it is possible to

Table 1
Prevalence of the anterolateral ligament in cadaveric studies

Investigators	Prevalence (%)	Population	Cadaver	Specimens (n°)	Pairing	Age (y)
Claes et al,[1] 2013	98	Belgian	Embalmed	41	Unpaired	79
Helito et al,[23] 2013	100	Brazilian	Fresh-frozen	20	Unpaired	61
Dodds et al,[22] 2014	83	British	Fresh-frozen	40	Unpaired	75
Caterine et al,[21] 2015	100	NA	Fresh-frozen	19	Paired/unpaired	70
Stijak et al,[29] 2016	50	Serbian	Embalmed	14	Unpaired	78
Kosy et al,[44] 2015	91	NA	Fresh-frozen	11	Unpaired	79
Runer et al,[28] 2016	45	Austrian	Embalmed	50	Unpaired	78
Roessler et al,[27] 2016	60	NA	Fresh-frozen	20	Paired	79
Potu et al,[26] 2016	4	White	Embalmed	24	Unpaired	NA
Watanabe et al,[30] 2016	37	Japanese	Embalmed	94	Unpaired/paired	86
Parker & Smith,[25] 2016	96	American	Embalmed	53	Unpaired/paired	67
Shea et al,[20] 2016	64	American	Fresh-frozen	14	Unpaired	8
Helito et al,[34] 2016	100	Brazilian	Embalmed	20	Unpaired	Fetus
Sabzevari et al,[19] 2017	0	American	Fresh-frozen	21	Unpaired	Fetus

Abbreviation: NA, not assessed.

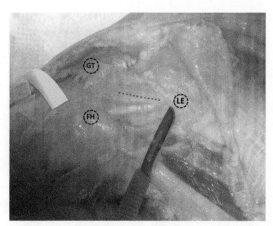

Fig. 1. With the iliotibial band reflected the cadaveric knee specimen is flexed. With internal rotation (*yellow arrow*) of the tibia the taut fibers of the anterolateral ligament (*red arrowheads*) can be seen running from the lateral epicondyle (LE) of the femur and inserting midway between the fibular head (FH) and the Gerdy tubercle (GT).

appreciate the ALL insertion more clearly, including its meniscal attachments.[31] Analysis of the numerous cadaveric studies has revealed a certain amount of variability in structure. The femoral origin of the ALL is typically found just posterior and proximal to the lateral epicondyle of the femur directly adhered to bone.[2] Its course is oblique, overlapping the proximal portion of the LCL, with some fibers attaching to the lateral meniscus and anterolateral capsule as it approaches the joint line. The tibial attachment is reported to be located around 1 cm below the joint line, midway between the fibular head and Gerdy tubercle[2] (**Fig. 2**). The ligament has been reported to be between 34 mm and 59 mm long, of variable thickness (nearly twice as thick in men compared with women), and to tighten with tibial internal rotation (**Fig. 3**).[2]

Careful review of the literature reveals several inconsistencies regarding certain anatomic features of the ALL. The femoral origin of the ALL has been described to

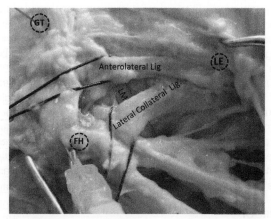

Fig. 2. Following sharp dissection it is possible to appreciate the anterolateral ligament as a separate structure from the joint capsule. Proximally the anterolateral ligament can be seen crossing superficial to the LCL. LM, lateral meniscus.

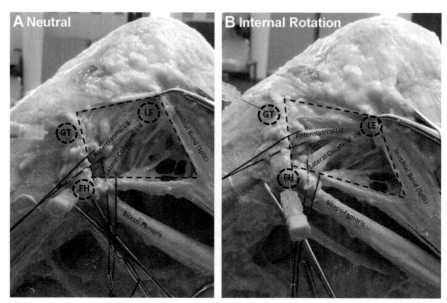

Fig. 3. In this specimen, in which the iliotibial band has been split at the level of the joint line (*dotted line*), it is possible to appreciate the anterolateral ligament (Lig.) tightening as the tibia is taken from a position of neutral rotation (*A*) to internal rotation (*B*).

be both anterior and distal and directly on the lateral epicondyle of the femur. The meniscal insertion has also been reported to be absent and changes in ligament length with knee flexion or extension have been variably reported.[1,22,32,33] These inconsistencies prevent the structure of the ALL from being characterized with certainty.

Considering the anatomic variability described, Helito and colleagues[34] proposed a theory of a multilayered ALL structure, identifying a superficial and deep ALL in 13 unpaired cadaveric knees. The superficial ALL inserted proximally and posteriorly with respect to the epicondyle, did not possess meniscal insertions, and increased its length with knee extension similar to previous reports by Dodds and colleagues[22] and Kennedy and colleagues.[32] In contrast, the deep ALL inserted in the center of the epicondyle, possessed insertions to lateral meniscus, and increased length with knee flexion, similar to previous reports by Claes and colleagues[1] and Zens and colleagues.[33] Although intriguing, the work of Helito and colleagues[34] is based on a small cadaveric sample and further studies are required.

In a recent roundtable discussion, a panel of experts was interrogated on the discrete nature of the ALL. Many panelists agreed that the ALL is a discrete ligamentous structure but others cited the capsulo-osseous layer of the iliotibial band described by Terry and colleagues[11] and the midthird capsular ligament described by Hughston and colleagues[7] as the main anterolateral knee structures in conjunction with the remainder of the ITB.[35,36] Based on these findings, similarities between the superficial ALL and the capsulo-ossous layer of the iliotibial band and between the deep ALL and the midthird capsular ligament have been suggested.[2,34]

ARTHROSCOPIC PROOF

Several investigators have suggested that it is possible to observe the ALL arthroscopically, describing a step-by-step procedure.[37,38] According to Zein,[38] the ALL can be visualized with a standard 30° arthroscope from a high anterolateral portal, with the knee in the figure-of-four position under varus stress. After entering the lateral gutter, the popliteal hiatus and the synovial bulge just anterior to the meniscal bare area (where the capsule reattaches to the meniscus) is identified. Advancing the arthroscope into the lateral gutter and on passing over the synovial bulge, the popliteus tendon, the LCL, and the ALL are seen in different planes, running in different directions. The ALL inserts proximally into the lateral aspect of the lateral femoral condyle, close to the popliteus and anterior to the LCL, whereas distally it inserts into the lateral aspect of the lateral meniscus anterior to the bare area. Applying internal rotation should show tightening the ALL, which can be probed. The meniscotibial attachment of the ALL can be seen and probed under the lateral meniscus, anterior to the popliteus tendon.

RADIOLOGICAL PROOF

The presence of the ALL has been supported by several imaging studies, in which both intact and injured ligaments have been described[21,39–47] (**Table 2**). Helito and colleagues[48] performed a surgical dissection of 13 unpaired knees previously evaluated with MRI, reporting an excellent correlation between anatomic and radiographic parameters of the ALL, including length, width, and distance from LCL and tibial plateau. On MRI, the ALL is best identified in the coronal plane, using proton density–weighted and T2-weighted sequences.[42] The ALL can be followed as a continuous band of low

Table 2
Prevalence of the anterolateral ligament and its features on MRI studies

Investigators	Subjects	Whole ALL (%)	Any Part (%)	Femoral Part	Tibial Part	Meniscal Part
Caterine et al,[21] 2014	10 cadavers	100	NA	Not clearly visible in many	Easily identified	Close relationship
Taneja et al,[46] 2015	70 knees	11	40	Not reliably seen	NA	0%
Porrino et al,[45] 2015	73 knees	100	NA	Inseparable from LCL	Inseparable from ITB	100%
Helito et al,[42] 2014	39 uninjured knees	71.7	97.8	89.7%	74.9%	94.8%
Kosy et al,[44] 2015	100 uninjured knees	57	94	59%	94%	94%
Helito et al,[41] 2015	33 uninjured knees	33.3	81.8	69.6%	39.3%	75.7%
Claes et al,[39] 2014	271 ACL-def knees	NA	76[a]	NA	NA	NA
Hartigan et al,[40] 2016	72 ACL-def knees	NA	100[a]	NA	NA	NA
Van Dyck et al,[47] 2016	90 ACL-def knees	NA	100[a]	NA	NA	NA
Helito et al,[43] 2017	101 ACL-def knees	NA	87.1[a]	NA	NA	NA

Abbreviation: def, deficient.
[a] Intact or injured ALL.

signal intensity from the lateral femoral epicondyle to the anterolateral tibia. A discrete proximal insertion is difficult to discern because of the proximity of the LCL. Along its distal course, deep to the iliotibial band, there is a more discrete meniscotibial component inserting below the level of the lateral tibial plateau midway between the fibular head and the Gerdy tubercle. Connections between the ALL and lateral meniscus have been reported consistently, with complete, central, bipolar, or inferior-only connection patterns.[44] In a series of patients with intact and ACL-deficient knees, the ALL was identified in up to 97.8% of the cases; lower percentages were reported in identifying the whole ALL or the single femoral, tibial, or meniscal part.[21,39–47] In contrast with these studies, Flores and colleagues[49] questioned whether the ALL can be identified on MRI. After analyzing 146 MRI studies of patients with a Segond fracture, they did not report other structures to be attached to the avulsed bone fragment except for what was defined by the investigators as the "meniscotibial component of the mid-third capsular ligament"[49] and "posterior fibers of the iliotibial band."[49]

Using ultrasonography, a structure identified as the ALL has been reported in both patient and cadaver studies. Oshima and colleagues[50] used real-time ultrasonography and found that the femoral and tibial portions but not the meniscal attachments of the ALL can be readily identified. Furthermore, Oshima and colleagues[50] measured the length and thickness of the ALL and found them to be similar to those in previous anatomic studies. In a similar study on 18 cadaveric knee specimens, Cavaignac and colleagues[51] identified the ALL with ultrasonography imaging, showing a good correlation with the anatomic findings obtained during subsequent anatomic dissection.

SUMMARY

In summary, historical, anatomic, and radiological evidence for the existence of the ALL is present. Despite this, because of inconsistencies in anatomic nomenclature, differences in dissection technique, and variability in cadaveric specimen characteristics, an agreement among experts regarding the description of the ALL as a distinct ligament cannot be reached. The anatomic course of the ALL remains a subject of controversy and ongoing study.

REFERENCES

1. Claes S, Vereecke E, Maes M, et al. Anatomy of the anterolateral ligament of the knee. J Anat 2013;223(4):321–8.
2. Sonnery-Cottet B, Daggett M, Fayard J-M, et al. Anterolateral Ligament Expert Group consensus paper on the management of internal rotation and instability of the anterior cruciate ligament - deficient knee. J Orthop Traumatol 2017. http://dx.doi.org/10.1007/s10195-017-0449-8.
3. Guenther D, Rahnemai-Azar AA, Bell KM, et al. The anterolateral capsule of the knee behaves like a sheet of fibrous tissue. Am J Sports Med 2017;45(4):849–55.
4. Musahl V, Rahnemai-Azar AA, Costello J, et al. The influence of meniscal and anterolateral capsular injury on knee laxity in patients with anterior cruciate ligament injuries. Am J Sports Med 2016;44(12):3126–31.
5. Musahl V, Rahnemai-Azar AA, van Eck CF, et al. Anterolateral ligament of the knee, fact or fiction? Knee Surg Sports Traumatol Arthrosc 2016;24(1):2–3.
6. Bänderlhre HJ. Handbuch Der Systematischen Anatomie Des Menschen, vol. 8. Braunscweig (Germany): Braunschweig; 1872.
7. Hughston JC, Andrews JR, Cross MJ, et al. Classification of knee ligament instabilities. Part II. The lateral compartment. J Bone Joint Surg Am 1976;58(2):173–9.

8. Jost A. Sur la morphogénèse et le rôle fonctionnel des ligaments épicondylo-méniscaux du genou. In: Compte Rendu de La Société de Biologie, vol. LXXXIV. 1921.

9. Müller W. The knee: form, function and ligament reconstruction. Berlin: Springer; 1982.

10. Segond P. Recherches cliniques et expérimentales sur les épanchements sanguins du genou par entorse. Progres Med 1879;7:297–341.

11. Terry GC, Hughston JC, Norwood LA. The anatomy of the iliopatellar band and iliotibial tract. Am J Sports Med 1986;14(1):39–45.

12. Vallois H. Etude Anatomique de L'articulation Du Genou Chez Les Primates. Montpellier: Abeille; 1914.

13. Weitbrecht J. Desmographie Ou Description Des Ligaments Du Corps Humain Avec Figures. Paris: Durand; 1752.

14. Vincent J-P, Magnussen RA, Gezmez F, et al. The anterolateral ligament of the human knee: an anatomic and histologic study. Knee Surg Sports Traumatol Arthrosc 2012;20(1):147–52.

15. Lubowitz JH, Provencher MT, Brand JC, et al. The knee anterolateral ligament. Arthroscopy 2014;30(11):1385–8.

16. Cavaignac E, Ancelin D, Chiron P, et al. Historical perspective on the "discovery" of the anterolateral ligament of the knee. Knee Surg Sports Traumatol Arthrosc 2016. http://dx.doi.org/10.1007/s00167-016-4349-x.

17. Ingham SJM, de Carvalho RT, Martins CAQ, et al. Anterolateral ligament anatomy: a comparative anatomical study. Knee Surg Sports Traumatol Arthrosc 2015. http://dx.doi.org/10.1007/s00167-015-3956-2.

18. Helito CP, do Prado Torres JA, Bonadio MB, et al. Anterolateral ligament of the fetal knee. Am J Sports Med 2017;45(1):91–6.

19. Sabzevari S, Rahnemai-Azar AA, Albers M, et al. Anatomic and histological investigation of the anterolateral capsular complex in the fetal knee. Am J Sports Med 2017. http://dx.doi.org/10.1177/0363546517692534.

20. Shea KG, Milewski MD, Cannamela PC, et al. Anterolateral ligament of the knee shows variable anatomy in pediatric specimens. Clin Orthop 2016. http://dx.doi.org/10.1007/s11999-016-5123-6.

21. Caterine S, Litchfield R, Johnson M, et al. A cadaveric study of the anterolateral ligament: re-introducing the lateral capsular ligament. Knee Surg Sports Traumatol Arthrosc 2015;23(11):3186–95.

22. Dodds AL, Halewood C, Gupte CM, et al. The anterolateral ligament: anatomy, length changes and association with the Segond fracture. Bone Joint J 2014; 96-B(3):325–31.

23. Helito CP, Demange MK, Bonadio MB, et al. Anatomy and histology of the knee anterolateral ligament. Orthop J Sports Med 2013;1(7). 2325967113513546.

24. Kosy JD, Soni A, Venkatesh R, et al. The anterolateral ligament of the knee: unwrapping the enigma. Anatomical study and comparison to previous reports. J Orthop Traumatol 2016;17(4):303–8.

25. Parker M, Smith HF. Anatomical variation in the anterolateral ligament of the knee and a new dissection technique for embalmed cadaveric specimens. Anat Sci Int 2016. http://dx.doi.org/10.1007/s12565-016-0386-2.

26. Potu BK, Salem AH, Abu-Hijleh MF. Morphology of anterolateral ligament of the knee: a cadaveric observation with clinical insight. Adv Med 2016;2016:9182863.

27. Roessler PP, Schüttler KF, Heyse TJ, et al. The anterolateral ligament (ALL) and its role in rotational extra-articular stability of the knee joint: a review of anatomy and surgical concepts. Arch Orthop Trauma Surg 2016;136(3):305–13.

28. Runer A, Birkmaier S, Pamminger M, et al. The anterolateral ligament of the knee: a dissection study. Knee 2016;23(1):8–12.

29. Stijak L, Bumbaširević M, Radonjić V, et al. Anatomic description of the anterolateral ligament of the knee. Knee Surg Sports Traumatol Arthrosc 2016;24(7): 2083–8.

30. Watanabe J, Suzuki D, Mizoguchi S, et al. The anterolateral ligament in a Japanese population: study on prevalence and morphology. J Orthop Sci 2016; 21(5):647–51.

31. Daggett M, Busch K, Sonnery-Cottet B. Surgical dissection of the anterolateral ligament. Arthrosc Tech 2016;5(1):e185–188.

32. Kennedy MI, Claes S, Fuso FAF, et al. The anterolateral ligament: an anatomic, radiographic, and biomechanical analysis. Am J Sports Med 2015;43(7): 1606–15.

33. Zens M, Niemeyer P, Ruhhammer J, et al. Length changes of the anterolateral ligament during passive knee motion: a human cadaveric study. Am J Sports Med 2015;43(10):2545–52.

34. Helito CP, do Amaral C, Nakamichi YD, et al. Why do authors differ with regard to the femoral and meniscal anatomic parameters of the knee anterolateral ligament?: dissection by layers and a description of its superficial and deep layers. Orthop J Sports Med 2016;4(12). 2325967116675604.

35. Herbst E, Albers M, Burnham JM, et al. The anterolateral complex of the knee: a pictorial essay. Knee Surg Sports Traumatol Arthrosc 2017. http://dx.doi.org/10. 1007/s00167-017-4449-2.

36. Musahl V, Getgood A, Neyret P, et al. Contributions of the anterolateral complex and the anterolateral ligament to rotatory knee stability in the setting of ACL injury: a roundtable discussion. Knee Surg Sports Traumatol Arthrosc 2017. http://dx. doi.org/10.1007/s00167-017-4436-7.

37. Sonnery-Cottet B, Archbold P, Rezende FC, et al. Arthroscopic identification of the anterolateral ligament of the knee. Arthrosc Tech 2014;3(3):e389–392.

38. Zein AMNE. Step-by-step arthroscopic assessment of the anterolateral ligament of the knee using anatomic landmarks. Arthrosc Tech 2015;4(6):e825–831.

39. Claes S, Bartholomeeusen S, Bellemans J. High prevalence of anterolateral ligament abnormalities in magnetic resonance images of anterior cruciate ligament-injured knees. Acta Orthop Belg 2014;80(1):45–9.

40. Hartigan DE, Carroll KW, Kosarek FJ, et al. Visibility of anterolateral ligament tears in anterior cruciate ligament-deficient knees with standard 1.5-tesla magnetic resonance imaging. Arthrosc J Arthrosc Relat Surg 2016;32(10):2061–5.

41. Helito CP, Demange MK, Helito PVP, et al. Evaluation of the anterolateral ligament of the knee by means of magnetic resonance examination. Rev Bras Ortop 2015; 50(2):214–9.

42. Helito CP, Helito PVP, Costa HP, et al. MRI evaluation of the anterolateral ligament of the knee: assessment in routine 1.5-T scans. Skeletal Radiol 2014;43(10): 1421–7.

43. Helito CP, Helito PVP, Costa HP, et al. Assessment of the anterolateral ligament of the knee by magnetic resonance imaging in acute injuries of the anterior cruciate ligament. Arthrosc J Arthrosc Relat Surg 2017;33(1):140–6.

44. Kosy JD, Mandalia VI, Anaspure R. Characterization of the anatomy of the anterolateral ligament of the knee using magnetic resonance imaging. Skeletal Radiol 2015;44(11):1647–53.

45. Porrino J, Maloney E, Richardson M, et al. The anterolateral ligament of the knee: MRI appearance, association with the Segond fracture, and historical perspective. AJR Am J Roentgenol 2015;204(2):367–73.
46. Taneja AK, Miranda FC, Braga CAP, et al. MRI features of the anterolateral ligament of the knee. Skeletal Radiol 2015;44(3):403–10.
47. Van Dyck P, Clockaerts S, Vanhoenacker FM, et al. Anterolateral ligament abnormalities in patients with acute anterior cruciate ligament rupture are associated with lateral meniscal and osseous injuries. Eur Radiol 2016;26(10):3383–91.
48. Helito CP, Helito PVP, Bonadio MB, et al. Correlation of magnetic resonance imaging with knee anterolateral ligament anatomy: a cadaveric study. Orthop J Sports Med 2015;3(12). 2325967115621024.
49. Flores DV, Smitaman E, Huang BK, et al. Segond fracture: an MR evaluation of 146 patients with emphasis on the avulsed bone fragment and what attaches to it. Skeletal Radiol 2016;45(12):1635–47.
50. Oshima T, Nakase J, Numata H, et al. Ultrasonography imaging of the anterolateral ligament using real-time virtual sonography. Knee 2016;23(2):198–202.
51. Cavaignac E, Wytrykowski K, Reina N, et al. Ultrasonographic identification of the anterolateral ligament of the knee. Arthrosc J Arthrosc Relat Surg 2016;32(1): 120–6.

Biomechanics of the Anterolateral Structures of the Knee

Christoph Kittl, MD[a], Eivind Inderhaug, MD, PhD[b],
Andy Williams, FRCS(Orth)[c], Andrew A. Amis, FREng, DSc[d,e],*

KEYWORDS

- Anterolateral • Tenodesis • Ligament • Iliotibial tract • Rotatory instability
- Pivot-shift

KEY POINTS

- The primary soft tissue restraint to tibial internal rotation has been found to be the deep layer of the iliotibial tract, connecting from Kaplan fibers on the femur to Gerdy's tubercle on the tibia.
- The anterolateral ligament has been found to be relatively weak and poorly aligned to resist tibial internal rotation, but damage here does increase laxity and may be a sign of other structures being damaged.
- Although lateral tenodeses are not anatomic, they are effective in controlling tibial internal rotation.

BACKGROUND

Previously, the term anterolateral rotatory instability (ALRI) was synonymous for the instability caused by an isolated anterior cruciate ligament (ACL) injury. Hughston and colleagues[1] were the first to popularize the idea that only a concomitant antero-lateral capsular injury can induce this excessive anterior subluxation of the lateral tibial

Disclosures: The authors declare that they have no conflicts of interest relating to this article. However, work that led up to this article was supported as follows: C. Kittl: AGA (Arthroscopy Association of the German-speaking countries); E. Inderhaug: Bergen Regional Health Authority; A. Williams and A.A. Amis: Smith & Nephew Co supported research studies at Imperial College London and educational lectures at conferences.
[a] Department of Trauma, Hand and Reconstructive Surgery, Westphalian Wilhelms University Muenster, Muenster DE 48149, Germany; [b] Orthopaedic Surgery Department, Haraldsplass Hospital, Bergen 5009, Norway; [c] Fortius Clinic, Fitzhardinge Street, London W1H 6EQ, UK; [d] Biomechanics Group, Mechanical Engineering Department, Imperial College London, London SW7 2AZ, UK; [e] Musculoskeletal Surgery Group, Imperial College School of Medicine, Charing Cross Hospital, London W6 8RF, UK
* Corresponding author. Biomechanics Group, Mechanical Engineering Department, Imperial College London, London SW7 2AZ, UK.
E-mail address: a.amis@imperial.ac.uk

Clin Sports Med 37 (2018) 21–31
http://dx.doi.org/10.1016/j.csm.2017.07.004
0278-5919/18/© 2017 Elsevier Inc. All rights reserved.

plateau. With the introduction of arthroscopic ACL surgery, these peripheral injuries fell out of focus. Although intra-articular reconstruction of the ACL restored knee kinematics in the anterior/posterior direction, it failed to completely abolish the pivot-shift phenomenon in some knees.[2] This led to a more anatomic approach of intra-articular ACL reconstruction, reproducing its oblique course to the posterior aspect of the femur by using the medial portal technique.[3] However, despite many efforts to improve tunnel positioning, graft tensioning, and after-care protocols, rotational laxity still has not been completely abolished.[4]

This residual rotational laxity after ACL reconstruction may come from additional injury of the peripheral structures, which gained broad interest after anatomic description of the anterolateral ligament (ALL) in 2013.[5] Since then, many studies regarding anatomy, biomechanics, and possible reconstructions have been conducted.[6–10] However, there is still a lack of evidence on how to diagnose these injuries and more importantly which patients will benefit from an additional lateral extra-articular procedure.

Although this work has given promising biomechanical and clinical results, these questions must be clarified by level I studies. Similar to the medial side, anterolateral capsular structures may have a high healing potential, when the primary restraint to anterior tibial translation is reconstructed, so routine use of anterolateral procedures may place the patient at unnecessary risk of an additional extra-articular procedure. Conversely, undiagnosed anterolateral structure injuries may "stretch-out" over time in chronic cases and impose abnormal loads on the ACL graft, preventing it from healing in the bone tunnel.[11] The purpose of this review was to provide a biomechanical rationale regarding the anterolateral structures of the knee.

ANATOMY OF THE ANTEROLATERAL STRUCTURES

The anatomy on the anterolateral side of the knee can best be described in a layer-by-layer fashion. The first relevant layer is the iliotibial tract (ITT), which inserts onto the tibia at the Gerdy's tubercle and extents proximally as the fascia lata, merging into the gluteus maximus, gluteus medius, and tensor fascia lata muscles. The second layer is formed by the posterior fiber region of the superficial tract, which merges with the deep and capsulo-osseous structures of the ITT (**Fig. 1**).[12]

The deep layer of the ITT becomes visible approximately 60 mm proximal to the lateral femoral epicondyle.[12] A triangular area at the distal termination of the lateral intermuscular septum is formed by strong fibers (Kaplan fibers) connecting the superficial ITT layer to the femur. The capsulo-osseous layer was described as the deepest layer of the ITT and provides a lateral capsular strengthening.[13] This layer is also known as the retrograde tract insertion[14] and attaches at the lateral femoral supracondylar region and passes distal, where it inserts slightly posterior to the Gerdy's tubercle. This ligament-like unit is composed of the deep and capsulo-osseous layers of the ITT, and forms a sling around the posterolateral aspect of the femur, inserting posterior to the Gerdy's tubercle and was described as "acting as an anterolateral ligament" by Terry and colleagues[12,15] (**Fig. 2**).

The next layer is formed by the mid-third lateral capsular ligament, which can be divided into a meniscotibial portion and a meniscofemoral portion.[1] On the tibia, it attaches between the anteroinferior popliteomeniscal fascicle (popliteus hiatus) and the posterior border of the Gerdy's tubercle approximately 6 to 9 mm distal from the joint line.[16–20] The femoral attachment site was defined in the region of the lateral femoral epicondyle[17,19] with several other attachments on the posterior aspect of the popliteus attachment and at the lateral gastrocnemius tendon attachment.[21]

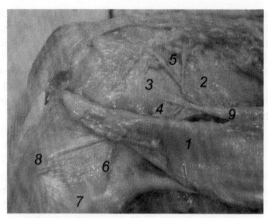

Fig. 1. Lateral aspect of a left knee. The superficial layer (1) of the iliotibial band (ITB) has been flapped down, revealing the Kaplan fibers. The lateral superior genicular artery (5) passes through the lateral intermuscular septum (9) between the proximal (2) and supracondylar insertion (3). The retrograde insertion (4; capsulo-osseous layer) forms a sling around the posterolateral femur and inserts distally somewhat posterior to the Gerdy's tubercle (8). Lateral collateral ligament (6); fibular head (7). (*From* Kittl C, El-Daou H, Athwal KK, et al. The role of the anterolateral structures and the ACL in controlling laxity of the intact and ACL-deficient knee. Am J Sports Med 2016;44:347; with permission.)

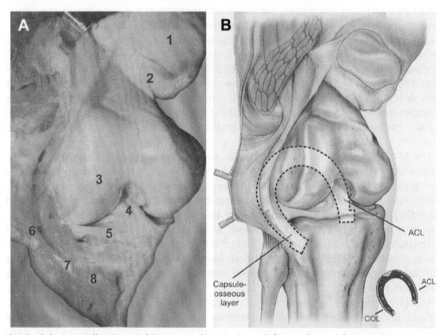

Fig. 2. (*A*) 1, patella; 2, quadriceps tendon; 3, lateral femoral condyle; 4, ACL; 5, lateral meniscus; 6, caspulo-osseous layer of the iliotibial band; 7, tibial insertion site of the capsulo-osseous layer; 8, Gerdy's tubercle. (*B*) The ACL and the capsulo-osseous layer (COL) of the ITB form a sling around the lateral femoral condyle. (*From* Vieira EL, Vieira EA, da Silva RT, et al. An anatomic study of the iliotibial tract. Arthroscopy 2007;23:273; with permission.)

The recently rediscovered ALL, first published by Vincent and colleagues,[10] does not really fit in this layered anatomy. Depending on the investigator, this ligament is either described as a capsular thickening or as part of the capsulo-osseous layer of the ITT. Claes and colleagues[5] described a capsular ligament with a femoral insertion on the tip of the lateral femoral epicondyle, which was present in 97% of their dissected knees, and an intermediate connection to the lateral meniscus was observed. Their description is similar to the mid-third lateral capsular ligament popularized by Hughston and colleagues.[1]

ANTEROLATERAL ROTATORY INSTABILITY OF THE KNEE

The ACL is the primary restraint to anterior tibial translation and the posterior cruciate ligament to posterior tibial translation.[22] It has been found that the tibia can be translated 30% more if it is free to rotate.[23] This "coupled" rotation in response to an anterior translation of the tibia results in a 3° to 10° internal rotation when examined by hand and slightly more in an ACL rupture. This is due to the more mobile lateral knee compartment, caused by the convex articular surfaces, the loose meniscocapsular attachment, and the less pronounced posterior wedge-effect of the relatively more mobile lateral meniscus.

From video analysis studies,[24] it is known that the trauma mechanism for noncontact ACL rupture involves a tibial internal rotational component. This is reinforced by the fact that the bone bruise found after a typical ACL rupture occurs at the posterolateral aspect of the tibia, which indicates this internal rotation movement.[25] In the actual injury situation, however, the abduction moment of the knee forces the lateral femoral condyle to slide posterior on the convex lateral tibial slope. This anterior subluxation of the lateral tibial plateau or the posterior subluxation of the femur, has been shown to put the ACL under excessive load, which may eventually cause the ACL rupture.[26] Although the central position of the ACL does not suggest a potential restraint to internal tibial rotation, it has been shown that it has a significant impact at early flexion angles. At these flexion angles, the tightening of the ACL forces the tibia to rotate externally and locks the knee at full extension. This principle of the "screw home" mechanism is lost in an ACL-deficient knee, leaving the tibia to rotate internally.[27]

The ACL rupture mechanism also implies stretching or rupturing of the anterolateral structures, which cross the anterolateral joint line and are oriented in an oblique direction similar to the ACL.[28] In the event of excessive anterior translation of the lateral tibial plateau, the anterolateral structures will have a much greater lever arm than the ACL to resist the combined anterior translation plus internal rotation motion. This is best shown by the Segond fracture, which is a bony avulsion of the lateral tibial rim caused by the anterolateral structures[29] (**Fig. 3**). A combined injury of the ACL and the anterolateral structures will therefore lead to a high-grade translatory (anterior translation) and rotatory (internal rotation) instability, which may induce a high-grade pivot-shift test.[28]

The pivot-shift test imitates this typical anterior subluxation mechanism of an ACL rupture and correlates best with functional and subjective patient outcome after ACL reconstruction.[30] However, due to different bony geometry, integrity of the anterolateral and medial soft tissues, and hip abduction, this test has a large interobserver and intraobserver variability.[31,32] Based on recent biomechanical data, one may speculate that this subluxation of the lateral tibial plateau will increase when additional anterolateral structure damage is present.[33] The reduction event in 30° to 60° of flexion, which is felt as the typical clunk, will then be pronounced similarly. In a clinical

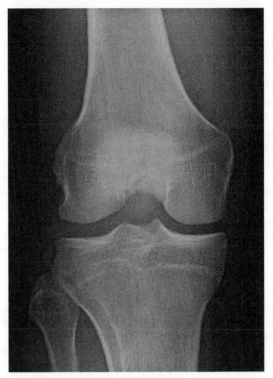

Fig. 3. Segond fracture (anterior-posterior radiograph).

pivot-shift testing setup, however, it seems difficult to distinguish between a normal and a high-grade pivot shift, because of the aforementioned variables. Thus, a specific clinical test to precisely identify ALRI is missing.

STRUCTURAL PROPERTIES OF THE ANTEROLATERAL STRUCTURES

When Werner Müller[34] dissected the lateral knee structures in his knee anatomy video for the European Society of Sports Traumatology, Knee Surgery and Arthroscopy, he mentioned one basic biomechanical principle: "Big structures, big function, small structures, small function." This does not necessarily mean that the bigger structures control anterior displacement of the lateral tibial plateau better than smaller structures. It strongly depends on fiber orientation (axis of alignment) to resist a certain displacement. The ITT, however, is tethered to the femoral metaphysis via the lateral intermuscular septum and the Kaplan fibers; therefore, the capsulo-osseous layer forms a sling around the posterolateral aspect of the lateral femoral condyle, implying a potent role in restraining anterior subluxation of the lateral tibial plateau.[13]

The ALL has been found to have a mean tensile strength of 49.9 to 319.7 N and a mean stiffness of 20 to 26 N/mm. These results come from differing descriptions of the anatomy of the ALL. Zens and colleagues[35] separated an isolated ALL structure, according to only one available anatomic article at this time, which had an ultimate strength of only 50 N. Other studies obviously included the capsulo-osseous layer of the iliotibial band (ITB), and found an ultimate tensile strength of 175 to 319 N and a mean stiffness of 20 to 26 N/mm.[36,37] This is similar to the structural properties of the deep medial collateral ligament (MCL), which is protected by the superficial fibers of the MCL,[38] like the anterolateral capsule and the deep fibers of the ITT are sheltered by the superficial ITT. Conversely, an 18-mm-wide strip of the ITT has been reported to have a mean tensile strength of 769 N.[39]

Length-Change Patterns of the Anterolateral Structures

In ligament surgery, the term isometry indicates the constant length of a graft during range of motion. From ACL reconstruction studies, we have learned that the effort to achieve true isometry will result in a nonanatomic graft placement, because isometry can apply only to a point-to-point connection and not to a graft or ligament attaching to an area of the bone.[40] This will cause different length-change patterns for different fiber regions. To reduce excessive length changes at each end of an attachment area, a flat ligament like the ACL and the superficial MCL will be twisted about its axis.[41] It also has been shown that isometry depends more on the femoral attachment than the tibial attachment.

It seems logical that the area at the axis of knee flexion, the transepicondylar axis, will be near to isometric, because the posterior aspects of the femoral condyles are almost spherical. However, due to the knee's roll-glide mechanism, the lateral condyle rolls posteriorly on the increasing posterior tibial slope. This makes it impossible to find a perfect isometric tibiofemoral connection, which has been shown by Sidles and colleagues.[42] They also found that a structure attaching anterior to the epicondyle will stretch with knee flexion, whereas structures attaching posterior to the epicondyle will slacken with knee flexion.

Looking at the ALL, 2 different attachment areas have been described. Vincent and colleagues[10] and Claes and colleagues[5] described an insertion area of the ALL anterior to and at the epicondyle, whereas several other studies[8,37] described an attachment area proximal and posterior to the epicondyle. The anterior attachment ALL has been found to increase in length from 0° to 90° of flexion by almost 20%.[43] This, however, means that it cannot be tight at early flexion angles and only control laxity at higher flexion angles. Conversely, the ALL, which attaches posterior to the epicondyle, may control laxity only at early flexion angle, and then slacken with knee flexion. This principle of the knee capsule also applies to the ITB, which can be divided into anterior and posterior fiber regions that act reciprocally. The posterior fiber region is tight in extension, whereas the anterior fiber region is tight in flexion (**Fig. 4**). The separation distance of the posterior attachment also has been measured by Dodds and colleagues,[8] by threading a suture along the ligament fibers attaching it to the tibia and a transducer. If the tibia was rotated internally, the separation distance increased (that is, the structure was stretched, causing tension to resist the tibial motion), whereas external rotation decreased the separation distance. Thus, anterolateral structures attaching posterior to the lateral femoral epicondyle are tight in early flexion angles and, due to their oblique course, are able to restrain the anterior subluxation of the lateral tibial plateau.

CONFUSION SURROUNDING THE ROLE OF THE ANTEROLATERAL STRUCTURES

Hughston and colleagues[1] were the first to popularize the term "anterolateral rotatory instability" and associated it with a rupture of the mid-third lateral capsular ligament and the ACL. However, they did not mention the capsulo-osseous layer of the ITT, which obviously runs directly above the anterolateral knee capsule. Terry and colleagues[15] and later Vieira and colleagues,[13] described the capsulo-osseous layer of the ITT forming a sling around the posterolateral femur and called it the "anterolateral

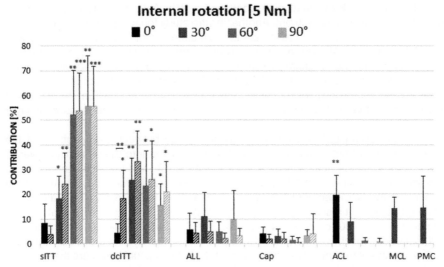

Fig. 4. Contribution of the anterolateral structures in controlling a 5 Nm internal rotation torque at 0°, 30°, 60°, and 90° of knee flexion. Cross-hatched areas indicate results from the ACL-deficient knee (n = 8). Together the superficial fibers (sITT) and the deep fibers (dcITT) of the ITT present the primary restraint to internal rotation at 30° to 90° of flexion. Conversely, the ALL and the anterolateral capsule (Cap) show a nonsignificant contribution in restraining internal rotation. MCL, n = 4; PMC, n = 4; *P<.05; **P<.01; ***P<.001. (*From* Kittl C, El-Daou H, Athwal KK, et al. The role of the anterolateral structures and the ACL in controlling laxity of the intact and ACL-deficient knee. Am J Sports Med 2016;44:350; with permission.)

ligament" (see **Fig. 3**). This was implied to resist anterolateral rotatory instability and was found to have been ruptured in 93% of the functionally unstable knees that they reconstructed. This fits with the observation of Terry and Laprade[44] that not only capsular structures insert at the Segond fracture, but also the capsulo-osseous layer of the ITB and the anterior arm of the biceps femoris muscle.

Recently there has been much confusion regarding the anatomy of the anterolateral structures. A distinct structure running distally across the anterolateral joint line from the lateral femoral epicondyle was described by Vincent and colleagues[10] in 2011 and later popularized by Claes and colleagues.[5] Since then, many articles described the ALL as a capsular or extra-capsular structure. Some of them claimed that the capsulo-osseous layer of the ITB and the ALL are the same structure and should be termed the anterolateral complex, similar to the posterolateral corner. However, in our own observations, we found a clear layer-by-layer anatomy existing of the superficial ITT layer, the deep and capsulo-osseous layer of the ITT, and the anterolateral capsule. In fact, in some knees, some fibers separated superficially from the capsular layer, such that they passed superficial to the lateral collateral ligament, and were so pronounced that they formed a capsular thickening imitating a distinct ligament. This observation is in line with several other studies, which did not find a distinct ligament on the anterolateral side in fresh frozen knees, formalin-embedded knees,[45] and fetal knees.[46]

There have been several cutting studies of the anterolateral side of the knee using a six degrees-of-freedom robotic setup, and almost all reported a significant increase in laxity after cutting the ALL. Parsons and colleagues[47] found a 30% to 45% contribution in restraining a 5-Nm internal rotation moment in 35° to 90° of knee flexion, falling to 5% near extension. Unfortunately, the ITB had been removed before testing;

therefore, most likely overstating the contribution of the ALL, as the ITB has since been shown to be the primary restraint. Another in vitro study found a pooled laxity increase of 2.8° of internal rotation in response to a simulated pivot shift, when the ALL was cut.[48] They cut the ALL on the tibia midway between the Gerdy's tubercle and the fibular head (Segond location), which has been found to be the attachment site for the capsulo-osseous ITB layer and the anterolateral capsular structures. Thus, most likely this increase in laxity did not only come from the ALL, but also from the combined transection of the whole anterolateral structures, including the capsulo-osseous layer of the ITT.

Kittl and colleagues[33] were the first to distinguish between the functions of the different layers of anterolateral structures, dividing them into the superficial layer of the ITT, the deep and capsulo-osseous layer of the ITT, and the capsular structures running superficial (ALL) and deep to the lateral collateral ligament (LCL; anterolateral capsule) in the ACL intact and ACL-deficient knee. They found that the ITT was the primary restraint (ie, it resisted more than 50% of the torque) to a 5-Nm internal rotation moment in 30° to 90° of flexion (see **Fig. 4**). The ACL had a significant contribution at full extension, which was taken by the capsulo-osseous layer of the ITT in the ACL-deficient state of the knee. Considering the ALL as the capsular structure that runs superficial to the LCL, it had only a minor role in resisting tibial internal rotation. However, these in vitro robotic studies present a scientific basis that can represent the "time-zero" situation only immediately after surgery, and the ultimate goal would be to measure rotational laxity in a weight-bearing situation or with a real-world injury.

Hudson and colleagues[49] reported that, in a normally aligned leg, walking caused tibial internal rotations of 13° during the stance phase. The axis of tibial internal-external rotation is close to the center of the tibial plateau when the soft tissues are intact,[50] so the peripheral capsular and overlying tissues will then be subjected to a shearing effect of approximately 10 to 12 mm, as the rim of the tibial plateau moves in relation to the outer surface of the femur. This movement will cause elongation of any soft tissue structure that crosses the joint line, if it had an orientation slanting in the correct direction (for example, on the lateral aspect, the tissue will be stretched by tibial internal rotation if the tibial attachment is anterior to the femoral attachment; and vice-versa on the medial aspect). Elongation of soft tissues leads to an elastic stretching response, and so they then resist the relative movement between the ends of the bones by increasing their tensile forces as the attachments move apart.

When Kittl and colleagues[33] used a robot to measure the contributions to resisting tibial internal rotation with the soft tissues intact, they reported that, at 30° knee flexion, the superficial ITB resisted 18% of the torque imposed on the tibia, the deep ITB 26%, the ALL 11%, the anterolateral (AL) capsule 3%, the ACL 9%, the MCL 15%, and the posteromedial capsule (PMC) 15%. Thus, the ITB resisted 44% and the ALL and AL capsule together resisted 14%, a total of 58%. Similarly, the MCL plus PMC resisted 30%. Thus, with the 9% of the ACL, we approach 100% of the resistance to tibial internal rotation arising solely from the soft tissues crossing the joint, and so almost none from the engagement of the articular surfaces and menisci, in this non–load-bearing test setup. The situation will differ under the loads encountered during gait, but there has been little work on rotation of the load-bearing knee.

SUMMARY

Tibial internal rotation is controlled mostly by the lateral extra-articular structures, which are the lateral capsule and the iliotibial band. Based on recent findings, the

ITT is the primary restraint to internal tibial rotation and the pivot-shift phenomenon as the knee flexes. The ALL is a capsular thickening, which has, similar to the deep MCL, only a secondary role in restraining the anterior subluxation of the lateral tibial plateau.

REFERENCES

1. Hughston J, Andrews J, Cross M, et al. Classification of knee ligament instabilities. Part II. The lateral compartment. J Bone Joint Surg Am 1976;58:173–9.
2. Lie DT, Bull AM, Amis AA. Persistence of the mini pivot shift after anatomically placed anterior cruciate ligament reconstruction. Clin Orthop Relat Res 2007; 457:203–9.
3. Harner CD, Honkamp NJ, Ranawat AS. Anteromedial portal technique for creating the anterior cruciate ligament femoral tunnel. Arthroscopy 2008;24: 113–5.
4. Sonnery-Cottet B, Thaunat M, Freychet B, et al. Outcome of a combined anterior cruciate ligament and anterolateral ligament reconstruction technique with a minimum 2-year follow-up. Am J Sports Med 2015;43:1598–605.
5. Claes S, Vereecke E, Maes M, et al. Anatomy of the anterolateral ligament of the knee. J Anat 2013;223:321–8.
6. Caterine S, Litchfield R, Johnson M, et al. A cadaveric study of the anterolateral ligament: re-introducing the lateral capsular ligament. Knee Surg Sports Traumatol Arthrosc 2015;23:3186–95.
7. Daggett M, Ockuly AC, Cullen M, et al. Femoral origin of the anterolateral ligament: an anatomic analysis. Arthroscopy 2016;32:835–41.
8. Dodds A, Halewood C, Gupte C, et al. The anterolateral ligament anatomy, length changes and association with the Segond fracture. Bone Joint J 2014;96:325–31.
9. Helito CP, Demange MK, Bonadio MB, et al. Anatomy and histology of the knee anterolateral ligament. Orthop J Sports Med 2013;1(7). 2325967113513546.
10. Vincent J-P, Magnussen RA, Gezmez F, et al. The anterolateral ligament of the human knee: an anatomic and histologic study. Knee Surg Sports Traumatol Arthrosc 2012;20:147–52.
11. Carson WG Jr. Extra-articular reconstruction of the anterior cruciate ligament: lateral procedures. Orthop Clin North Am 1985;16:191–211.
12. Terry GC, Hughston JC, Norwood LA. The anatomy of the iliopatellar band and iliotibial tract. Am J Sports Med 1986;14:39–45.
13. Vieira EL, Vieira EA, da Silva RT, et al. An anatomic study of the iliotibial tract. Arthroscopy 2007;23:269–74.
14. Lobenhoffer P, Posel P, Witt S, et al. Distal femoral fixation of the iliotibial tract. Arch Orthop Trauma Surg 1987;106:285–90.
15. Terry GC, Norwood LA, Hughston JC, et al. How iliotibial tract injuries of the knee combine with acute anterior cruciate ligament tears to influence abnormal anterior tibial displacement. Am J Sports Med 1993;21:55–60.
16. Reid JS, Van Slyke MA, Moulton MJ, et al. Safe placement of proximal tibial transfixation wires with respect to intracapsular penetration. J Orthop Trauma 2001;15: 10–7.
17. LaPrade RF, Gilbert TJ, Bollom TS, et al. The magnetic resonance imaging appearance of individual structures of the posterolateral knee. A prospective study of normal knees and knees with surgically verified grade III injuries. Am J Sports Med 2000;28:191–9.

18. Birrer S. The popliteus tendon and its fascicles at the popliteal hiatus: gross anatomy and functional arthroscopic evaluation with and without anterior cruciate ligament deficiency. Arthroscopy 1990;6:209–20.
19. Sanchez AR 2nd, Sugalski MT, LaPrade RF. Anatomy and biomechanics of the lateral side of the knee. Sports Med Arthrosc 2006;14:2–11.
20. Seebacher JR, Inglis AE, Marshall JL, et al. The structure of the posterolateral aspect of the knee. J Bone Joint Surg Am 1982;64:536–41.
21. LaPrade RF. Posterolateral knee injuries: anatomy, evaluation, and treatment. Stuggart (Germany): Thieme; 2006.
22. Butler DL, Noyes FR, Grood ES. Ligamentous restraints to anterior-posterior drawer in the human knee. A biomechanical study. J Bone Joint Surg Am 1980;62:259–70.
23. Amis AA, Bull AM, Lie DT. Biomechanics of rotational instability and anatomic anterior cruciate ligament reconstruction. Oper Tech Orthop 2005;15:29–35.
24. Olsen O-E, Myklebust G, Engebretsen L, et al. Injury mechanisms for anterior cruciate ligament injuries in team handball a systematic video analysis. Am J Sports Med 2004;32:1002–12.
25. Herbst E, Hoser C, Tecklenburg K, et al. The lateral femoral notch sign following ACL injury: frequency, morphology and relation to meniscal injury and sports activity. Knee Surg Sports Traumatol Arthrosc 2015;23:2250–8.
26. Kanamori A, Woo SL, Ma CB, et al. The forces in the anterior cruciate ligament and knee kinematics during a simulated pivot shift test: a human cadaveric study using robotic technology. Arthroscopy 2000;16:633–9.
27. Hallen L, Lindahl O. The "screw-home" movement in the knee-joint. Acta Orthop Scand 1966;37:97–106.
28. Wroble RR, Grood ES, Cummings JS, et al. The role of the lateral extraarticular restraints in the anterior cruciate ligament-deficient knee. Am J Sports Med 1993;21:257–63.
29. Claes S, Luyckx T, Vereecke E, et al. The Segond fracture: a bony injury of the anterolateral ligament of the knee. Arthrosc 2014;30:1475–82.
30. Kocher MS, Steadman JR, Briggs KK, et al. Relationships between objective assessment of ligament stability and subjective assessment of symptoms and function after anterior cruciate ligament reconstruction. Am J Sports Med 2004; 32:629–34.
31. Noyes FR, Grood ES, Cummings JF, et al. An analysis of the pivot shift phenomenon: the knee motions and subluxations induced by different examiners. Am J Sports Med 1991;19:148–55.
32. Bull AM, Andersen HN, Basso O, et al. Incidence and mechanism of the pivot shift: an in vitro study. Clin Orthop Relat Res 1999;363:219–31.
33. Kittl C, El-Daou H, Athwal KK, et al. The role of the anterolateral structures and the ACL in controlling laxity of the intact and ACL-deficient knee. Am J Sports Med 2016;44:345–54.
34. Müller W. Anatomy of the knee. Luxembourg: ESSKA; 2006.
35. Zens M, Feucht MJ, Ruhhammer J, et al. Mechanical tensile properties of the anterolateral ligament. J Exp Orthop 2015;2:7.
36. Rahnemai-Azar AA, Miller RM, Guenther D, et al. Structural properties of the anterolateral capsule and iliotibial band of the knee. Am J Sports Med 2016;44: 892–7.
37. Spencer L, Burkhart TA, Tran MN, et al. Biomechanical analysis of simulated clinical testing and reconstruction of the anterolateral ligament of the knee. Am J Sports Med 2015;43:2189–97.

38. Robinson JR, Bull AM, Amis AA. Structural properties of the medial collateral ligament complex of the human knee. J Biomech 2005;38:1067–74.
39. Noyes FR, Butler D, Grood E, et al. Biomechanical analysis of human ligament grafts used in knee-ligament repairs and reconstructions. J Bone Joint Surg Am 1984;66:344–52.
40. Zavras T, Race A, Bull A, et al. A comparative study of "isometric" points for anterior cruciate ligament graft attachment. Knee Surg Sports Traumatol Arthrosc 2001;9:28–33.
41. Müller W. Das Knie: form, Funktion und ligamentäre Wiederherstellungschirurgie. Heidelberg (Germany): Springer-Verlag; 2013.
42. Sidles JA, Larson RV, Garbini JL, et al. Ligament length relationships in the moving knee. J Orthop Res 1988;6:593–610.
43. Kittl C, Halewood C, Stephen JM, et al. Length change patterns in the lateral extra-articular structures of the knee and related reconstructions. Am J Sports Med 2015;43:354–62.
44. Terry GC, LaPrade RF. The biceps femoris muscle complex at the knee. Its anatomy and injury patterns associated with acute anterolateral-anteromedial rotatory instability. Am J Sports Med 1996;24:2–8.
45. Fardin PBA, Lizardo JHdF, Baptista JdS. Study of the anterolateral ligament of the knee in formalin-embedded cadavers. Acta Ortop Bras 2017;25(2):89–92.
46. Sabzevari S, Rahnemai-Azar AA, Albers M, et al. Anatomic and histological investigation of the anterolateral capsular complex in the fetal knee. Am J Sports Med 2017;45(6):1383–7.
47. Parsons EM, Gee AO, Spiekerman C, et al. The biomechanical function of the anterolateral ligament of the knee. Am J Sports Med 2015;43(3):669–74.
48. Rasmussen MT, Nitri M, Williams BT, et al. An in vitro robotic assessment of the anterolateral ligament, part 1: secondary role of the anterolateral ligament in the setting of an anterior cruciate ligament injury. Am J Sports Med 2016;44(3):585–92.
49. Hudson D, Royer T, Richards J. Bone mineral density of the proximal tibia relates to axial torsion in the lower limb. Gait Posture 2007;26(3):446–51.
50. Matsumoto H. Mechanism of the pivot shift. J Bone Joint Surg Br 1990;72-B:816–21. Accessed 2013-11-25 11:55:16.

Biomechanical Proof for the Existence of the Anterolateral Ligament

 CrossMark

Jorge Chahla, MD, PhD[a], Andrew G. Geeslin, MD[a],
Mark E. Cinque, MS[a], Robert F. LaPrade, MD, PhD[a,b],*

KEYWORDS

• Anterolateral ligament • Knee • Biomechanics • Rotational instability

KEY POINTS

- Awareness of the contribution of the anterolateral knee for rotational stability has reemerged in the literature.
- Improved understanding of the anatomy has led to an expansion of the literature on the biomechanics of the anterolateral knee, including the participation of the anterolateral ligament, as well as the iliotibial band, including the deep (Kaplan) fibers and the capsulo-osseous layer.
- The anterolateral ligament (ALL) resists tibial internal rotation at increased knee flexion angles, with a minimal role in anteroposterior stability.
- The contribution of other anterolateral structures has received less recent attention in the literature.
- Combined anatomic anterior cruciate ligament reconstruction (ACLR) and ALL reconstruction reduces tibial internal rotation compared with isolated ACLR with ALL deficiency, although may be associated with overconstraint.

INTRODUCTION

Although anterior cruciate ligament (ACL) reconstruction is one of the most common knee procedures, with more than 200,000 performed annually in the United States,[1,2] rotational instability persists in up to 25% of patients.[3] In patients with rotational laxity, tunnel positioning has often been deemed satisfactory, suggesting that successful treatment of these patients may be dependent on more than this factor alone. Several extra-articular techniques have emerged in the past 50 years to address rotational

R.F. LaPrade is a consultant and receives royalties from Arthrex, Össur, and Smith and Nephew.
[a] Steadman Philippon Research Institute, 181 West Meadow Drive, Suite 400, Vail, CO 81657, USA; [b] The Steadman Clinic, 181 West Meadow Drive, Suite 400, Vail, CO 81657, USA
* Corresponding author. Steadman Philippon Research Institute, The Stedman Clinic, 181 West Meadow Drive, Suite 400, Vail, CO 81657.
E-mail address: drlaprade@sprivail.org

Clin Sports Med 37 (2018) 33–40
http://dx.doi.org/10.1016/j.csm.2017.07.003
0278-5919/18/© 2017 Elsevier Inc. All rights reserved.

laxity in the setting of an ACL tear, primarily relying on augmenting or reconstructing the anterolateral structures of the knee. However, concerns of knee overconstraint with reconstruction of extra-articular structures have been raised, as overconstraint has been demonstrated in several biomechanical studies, and may lead to accelerated degenerative changes or ACL graft failure.[4–7]

Historically, the existence of an isolated ACL tear was infrequent and it was suspected that there were likely concomitant injuries to extra-articular stabilizing structures. Specifically, the anterolateral structures may be injured concomitantly with the ACL tear. For example, Helito and colleagues[8] evaluated the prevalence of anterolateral ligament (ALL) injury in 88 knees with an ACL tear and an identifiable ALL; 33 patients had imaging findings consistent with an injury to the ALL. Similar associated injury patterns also have been reported for the iliotibial band (ITB).[9] Failing to recognize these injuries at the time of ACL reconstruction may result in residual rotational laxity (pivot shift), a scenario that can potentially compromise the ACL graft. In fact, it has been suggested that an ALL reconstruction may be indicated in patients with chronic ACL tears, as well as those with a high-grade pivot shift.[10]

Recent studies have identified several structures likely to play a role in rotational stability, including the ALL,[11] the ITB,[12] and the lateral meniscus posterior root.[13] Much of the recent literature has focused on the anatomy and biomechanics of the ALL, and several reconstruction techniques have been described. The roles of key anterolateral knee structures are reviewed, with a specific emphasis on the anterolateral ligament, to improve the understanding of the influence of the anterolateral knee on rotational stability.

NOMENCLATURE AND ANATOMIC CONSIDERATIONS

A leading cause for an incomplete understanding of the biomechanical role of anterolateral knee structures is the inconsistency in anatomic descriptions and nomenclature. No consensus exists currently, as several investigators have provided different anatomic and functional descriptions, and heterogeneity in nomenclature has persisted.

In 1879, Segond[14] described an avulsion fracture of the proximal aspect of the anterolateral tibia that was subsequently reported to be associated with ACL injuries.[15,16] Additionally, he reported the existence of a structure that was associated with these lesions, which according to his description, was a pearly band extending in an oblique fashion from the femur inserting into the avulsed tibial bone. Interestingly, this description coincides with a capsular thickening of what Hughston and colleagues[17–19] termed the "mid-third lateral capsular ligament"[9] and also the anterior oblique band of the lateral collateral ligament described by Johnson.[20] Furthermore, Terry and colleagues,[18] in 1986, reported that the deep, capsulo-osseous and superficial layers of the iliotibial tract functioned as an "anterolateral ligament of the knee." Additionally, in 2007 Vieira and colleagues[21] reported that the capsulo-osseous layer acts as a "true" anterolateral ligament. Later, in 2013, Claes[22] described a reportedly distinct anatomic structure with well-defined anatomic attachments, which he termed "the anterolateral ligament of the knee." This more recent change in terminology was likely engendered by strong lay press-driven research studies, which validated the role of the ALL in anterior and rotational stability about the knee.[23]

BIOMECHANICAL ROLE OF KEY ANTEROLATERAL STRUCTURES

Several anterolateral knee structures likely contribute to restraining internal rotation, including the ALL, the superficial layer of the ITB, the ITB deep (Kaplan) fibers, the capsulo-osseous layer of the ITB, and the mid-third lateral capsular ligament.[19] It is suspected that the ALL may not be the sole extra-articular contributor to rotational stability. In this regard, there is some agreement regarding the ALL and its role in knee stability. Parsons and colleagues[23] reported that ALL restrains internal rotation at knee flexion of 35° or greater, with a minimal role in anteroposterior stability. Similarly, Rasmussen and colleagues[24] reported that the ALL had an important role for restraining internal rotation in ACL-deficient knees, especially at high flexion angles.

Recently, in an effort to determine the role of each of the anterolateral structures and the ACL in restraining simulated clinical laxity, Kittl and colleagues[25] reported that the ITB was the main extra-articular contributor to restraint of tibial internal rotation and anterior translation. Although several biomechanical studies have reported that the ALL is important in controlling internal rotation in ACL-deficient knees (**Fig. 1**),[23,24,26] Kittl and colleagues[25] reported that the ALL had only a minor role in controlling internal rotation in ACL-deficient knees. Sonnery-Cottet and colleagues[26] reported that both the ITB and the ALL have a significant role in controlling internal rotation at 20° and 90°, and coupled axial rotation during a pivot shift, with the ITB contributing more to restraining internal rotation. From this, it can be postulated that the anterolateral knee structures act synergistically in controlling internal rotation at higher flexion angles.

The distal ITB deep (Kaplan) fibers have been reported to act as a stabilizing ligament (**Fig. 2**), securing the distal portion of the ITB against the lateral epicondyle

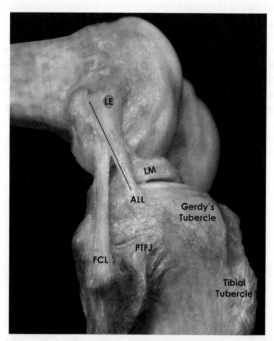

Fig. 1. Anatomic dissection demonstrating the course of the ALL in a right knee cadaveric specimen. The proximal attachment is located posterior and proximal to the FCL attachment. Of note, the ALL crosses the FCL superficially and inserts distally into the tibia approximately midway between the center of the Gerdy tubercle and the anterior margin of the fibular head. FCL, fibular collateral ligament; LE, lateral epicondyle; LM, lateral meniscus; PTFJ, proximal tibiofibular joint.

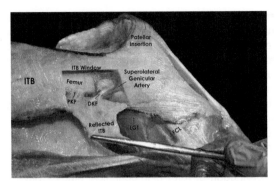

Fig. 2. Photograph of a right lateral femur specimen demonstrating the attachments of the proximal (PKF) and distal Kaplan fibers (DKF) and their relationship with the superolateral genicular artery. LGT, lateral gastrocnemius tendon; PLT, popliteus tendon.

and increasing in tension during internal rotation.[27] Terry and colleagues[9] and Yamamoto and colleagues[28] reported that the ITB was the key structure in controlling the anterolateral rotational instability (pivot-shift maneuver). Injuries to the ITB were identified in 93% of the patients, and a correlation was described between these injuries and a positive pivot-shift test, anterior tibial translation at 90°, and the Lachman test.[9] Similarly, in a biomechanical study on cadaveric knees, Yamamoto and colleagues[28] reported on the important role of the ITB in controlling coupled anterior tibial translation during a simulated pivot-shift test at high flexion angles.

The individual roles of the capsulo-osseous layer and the mid-third lateral capsular ligament are less understood because no sectioning studies have elucidated the contribution of each structure to rotational stability (**Fig. 3**). For example, in a cadaveric study, Wroble and colleagues[29] reported a significant increase in internal rotation at angles ≥30° after sectioning the "iliotibial band and midlateral structures." Because the individual roles of these structures were not specifically investigated, the influence of each structure could not be determined. Moreover, the prevalence of injury of these separate structures (concomitantly with ACL tears) has not been defined as of yet, making it challenging to assess the real contribution of the different anatomic structures.

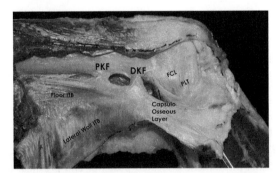

Fig. 3. Cadaveric dissection depicting the insertions of the PKF and DKF on the proximal and distal ridges of the lateral femur, respectively, in a right knee. A distinct fascial portion of the deep ITB, the capsulo-osseous layer, attaches just proximal to the lateral gastrocnemius tubercle, on the distal ridge and courses superficially to the FCL and PLT.

The ALL has been reported to be a key stabilizer to tibial internal rotatory stability. Its action is more prominent as the knee flexes past 30°.[23,30–32] However, in the clinical setting, residual rotational instability after ACL reconstruction in symptomatic patients occurs near extension and at up to 30° of knee flexion, and identified by a positive pivot-shift test during the physical examination. This suggests that the presence of other structures in the anterolateral knee act synergistically to prevent rotational instability.

Rasmussen and colleagues[24] reported that the presence of a combined ACL and ALL lesion caused the knee to have a significantly higher internal rotational instability and axial plane translation during the pivot-shift test when compared with an isolated ACL tear. Although a knee with a deficient ALL has a 1.7° to 1.8° increase in internal rotation laxity, a recent cadaveric study suggested that a concomitant ACL and ALL reconstruction further reduced rotatory laxity compared with isolated ACL reconstruction in knees with a combined ACL and ALL deficiency.[33] Isolated ACLR resulted in significant residual internal rotation compared with the fully intact knee during applied internal rotation torques and a simulated pivot shift in an ALL-deficient knee. By adding an ALL reconstruction in this study, internal rotation was significantly reduced and therefore comparable with the intact state.[33]

ANTEROLATERAL LIGAMENT RECONSTRUCTION

In 2 recent biomechanical analyses of ALL reconstruction, knee overconstraint was reported when using a posterior/proximal femoral ALL reconstruction tunnel.[11,33] However, other studies using the same femoral fixation point did not identify overconstraint after ALL reconstruction.[31,34] Furthermore, the latter studies did not report a significant difference between the ALL reconstructed and the ALL-deficient knee during internal rotation or pivot-shift testing.[31,34] This inability to restore internal rotation may have been secondary to low graft tensioning forces or the anterior femoral fixation of the ALL grafts.[31,34] These studies highlight a discrepancy between the biomechanical properties of the native structures and reconstruction procedures; the optimal reconstruction technique remains unclear.

Nitri and colleagues[33] studied the kinematics of ALL reconstruction in the setting of an ACL reconstruction, and compared intact and sectioned ALL states. The investigators reported that combined anatomic ACLR and ALL reconstruction improved rotatory stability of the knee compared with isolated ACLR with ALL deficiency. Similarly, Schon and colleagues[11] investigated the influence of knee flexion angles for graft fixation to identify an angle that would restore stability but not overconstrain the knee. The investigators reported that ALL reconstruction resulted in overconstraint at all fixation angles between 0 and 90° of knee flexion. Therefore, it was concluded that ALL reconstruction was unable to restore stability without overconstraining normal joint kinematics.

However, other studies have reported contrasting results. Spencer and colleagues[31] reported that ALL reconstruction using Fiber-tape (Arthrex, Naples, FL) did not significantly reduce internal rotation or anterior translation, and thus did not overconstrain knee kinematics. Similar, Tavlo and colleagues[34] reported no overconstraint following ALL reconstruction using the ALL reconstruction according to the anatomic attachments described by Claes and colleagues.[22] In their study, ALL sectioning resulted in a significant increase in internal rotation in the ACL-deficient knees. Reconstruction of the ALL in the ACL-deficient knees improved anterior stability; however, ALL reconstruction failed to improve internal rotation.[34]

SUMMARY

A broad knowledge of the anterolateral knee anatomy is vital to understand its biomechanics, better diagnose instability patterns, and to ultimately precisely reconstruct the relevant injured structures. The anterolateral corner of the knee comprises several structures that work in conjunction to provide rotational stability to the knee. However, the information regarding the role of each structure is not yet clear. Although the anterolateral ligament has been reported to be an important stabilizer of the anterolateral complex, its overall role in providing anterolateral or internal rotation stability, especially compared with the ITB, is still being investigated. Further studies are required to precisely determine the role of each structure and the effect of injury, with support from clinical data. This will help to identify the proper indications for reconstruction, and the optimal surgical technique.

REFERENCES

1. Buller LT, Best MJ, Baraga MG, et al. Trends in anterior cruciate ligament reconstruction in the United States. Orthop J Sports Med 2015;3(1). 2325967114563664.
2. Wilde J, Bedi A, Altchek DW. Revision anterior cruciate ligament reconstruction. Sports Health 2014;6(6):504–18.
3. Sonnery-Cottet B, Thaunat M, Freychet B, et al. Outcome of a combined anterior cruciate ligament and anterolateral ligament reconstruction technique with a minimum 2-year follow-up. Am J Sports Med 2015;43(7):1598–605.
4. Strum GM, Fox JM, Ferkel RD, et al. Intraarticular versus intraarticular and extraarticular reconstruction for chronic anterior cruciate ligament instability. Clin Orthop Relat Res 1989;(245):188–98.
5. Andrews JR, Sanders RA, Morin B. Surgical treatment of anterolateral rotatory instability. A follow-up study. Am J Sports Med 1985;13(2):112–9.
6. Benum P. Anterolateral rotary instability of the knee joint. Results after stabilization by extraarticular transposition of the lateral part of the patellar ligament. A preliminary report. Acta Orthop Scand 1982;53(4):613–7.
7. Amirault JD, Cameron JC, MacIntosh DL, et al. Chronic anterior cruciate ligament deficiency. Long-term results of MacIntosh's lateral substitution reconstruction. J Bone Joint Surg Br 1988;70(4):622–4.
8. Helito CP, Helito PV, Costa HP, et al. Assessment of the anterolateral ligament of the knee by magnetic resonance imaging in acute injuries of the anterior cruciate ligament. Arthroscopy 2016;33(1):140–6.
9. Terry GC, Norwood LA, Hughston JC, et al. How iliotibial tract injuries of the knee combine with acute anterior cruciate ligament tears to influence abnormal anterior tibial displacement. Am J Sports Med 1993;21(1):55–60.
10. Sonnery-Cottet B, Barbosa NC, Tuteja S, et al. Minimally invasive anterolateral ligament reconstruction in the setting of anterior cruciate ligament injury. Arthrosc Tech 2016;5(1):e211–5.
11. Schon JM, Moatshe G, Brady AW, et al. Anatomic anterolateral ligament reconstruction of the knee leads to overconstraint at any fixation angle. Am J Sports Med 2016;44(10):2546–56.
12. Huser LE, Noyes FR, Jurgensmeier D, et al. Anterolateral ligament and iliotibial band control of rotational stability in the anterior cruciate ligament-intact knee: defined by tibiofemoral compartment translations and rotations. Arthroscopy 2016;33(3):595–604.

13. Shybut TB, Vega CE, Haddad J, et al. Effect of lateral meniscal root tear on the stability of the anterior cruciate ligament-deficient knee. Am J Sports Med 2015;43(4):905–11.

14. Segond P. Recherches cliniques et expérimentales sur les épanchements sanguins du genou par entorse. Aux Bureaux du Progrès médical. Paris, France: V.A. Delahaye; 1879.

15. Hess T, Rupp S, Hopf T, et al. Lateral tibial avulsion fractures and disruptions to the anterior cruciate ligament. A clinical study of their incidence and correlation. Clin Orthop Relat Res 1994;(303):193–7.

16. Goldman AB, Pavlov H, Rubenstein D. The Segond fracture of the proximal tibia: a small avulsion that reflects major ligamentous damage. AJR Am J Roentgenol 1988;151(6):1163–7.

17. Hughston JC. Acute knee injuries in athletes. Clin Orthop 1962;23:114–33.

18. Terry GC, Hughston JC, Norwood LA. The anatomy of the iliopatellar band and iliotibial tract. Am J Sports Med 1986;14(1):39–45.

19. Hughston JC, Andrews JR, Cross MJ, et al. Classification of knee ligament instabilities. Part II. The lateral compartment. J Bone Joint Surg Am 1976;58(2): 173–9.

20. Johnson LL. Lateral capsular ligament complex: anatomical and surgical considerations. Am J Sports Med 1979;7(3):156–60.

21. Vieira EL, Vieira EA, da Silva RT, et al. An anatomic study of the iliotibial tract. Arthroscopy 2007;23(3):269–74.

22. Claes S, Vereecke E, Maes M, et al. Anatomy of the anterolateral ligament of the knee. J Anat 2013;223(4):321–8.

23. Parsons EM, Gee AO, Spiekerman C, et al. The biomechanical function of the anterolateral ligament of the knee. Am J Sports Med 2015;43(8):NP22.

24. Rasmussen MT, Nitri M, Williams BT, et al. An in vitro robotic assessment of the anterolateral ligament, part 1: secondary role of the anterolateral ligament in the setting of an anterior cruciate ligament injury. Am J Sports Med 2016;44(3): 585–92.

25. Kittl C, El-Daou H, Athwal KK, et al. The role of the anterolateral structures and the ACL in controlling laxity of the intact and ACL-deficient knee: response. Am J Sports Med 2016;44(4):Np15–8.

26. Sonnery-Cottet B, Lutz C, Daggett M, et al. The involvement of the anterolateral ligament in rotational control of the knee. Am J Sports Med 2016;44(5): 1209–14.

27. Lutz C, Sonnery-Cottet B, Niglis L, et al. Behavior of the anterolateral structures of the knee during internal rotation. Orthop Traumatol Surg Res 2015; 101(5):523–8.

28. Yamamoto Y, Hsu WH, Fisk JA, et al. Effect of the iliotibial band on knee biomechanics during a simulated pivot shift test. J Orthop Res 2006;24(5):967–73.

29. Wroble RR, Grood ES, Cummings JS, et al. The role of the lateral extraarticular restraints in the anterior cruciate ligament-deficient knee. Am J Sports Med 1993;21(2):257–62 [discussion: 263].

30. Kennedy MI, Claes S, Fuso FA, et al. The anterolateral ligament: an anatomic, radiographic, and biomechanical analysis. Am J Sports Med 2015;43(7): 1606–15.

31. Spencer L, Burkhart TA, Tran MN, et al. Biomechanical analysis of simulated clinical testing and reconstruction of the anterolateral ligament of the knee. Am J Sports Med 2015;43(9):2189–97.

32. Van der Watt L, Khan M, Rothrauff BB, et al. The structure and function of the anterolateral ligament of the knee: a systematic review. Arthroscopy 2015;31(3): 569–82.e563.
33. Nitri M, Rasmussen MT, Williams BT, et al. An in vitro robotic assessment of the anterolateral ligament, part 2: anterolateral ligament reconstruction combined with anterior cruciate ligament reconstruction. Am J Sports Med 2016;44(3): 593–601.
34. Tavlo M, Eljaja S, Jensen JT, et al. The role of the anterolateral ligament in ACL insufficient and reconstructed knees on rotatory stability: a biomechanical study on human cadavers. Scand J Med Sci Sports 2016;26(8):960–6.

Structural Properties of the Anterolateral Complex and Their Clinical Implications

⊙ CrossMark

Gerald A. Ferrer, BS[a,b], Daniel Guenther, MD[c],
Thierry Pauyo, MD, FRCSC[a,d], Elmar Herbst, MD[a,d],
Kanto Nagai, MD, PhD[a,d], Richard E. Debski, PhD[a,b,d],
Volker Musahl, MD[a,b,e,*]

KEYWORDS

- Anterolateral structures of the knee • Anterolateral ligament • Anterolateral capsule

KEY POINTS

- The entire anterolateral complex has an impact on rotatory and translational stability of the knee.
- Reconstruction methods need to be adapted based on pattern of injury and amount of rotatory knee instability.
- Further biomechanical analysis of the anterolateral complex would potentially help physicians determine precise surgical indication for individualized surgical treatment and improve patient surgical outcomes.

INTRODUCTION

Advances in understanding of rotatory knee instability have been largely driven by the anterior cruciate ligament (ACL) injury and reconstruction.[1–3] The anterolateral complex works together with the ACL to control rotation of the knee and is a secondary restraint to internal tibial rotation. In most typical descriptions, the anterolateral complex contains the superficial and deep iliotibial band (ITB), the capsulo-osseous layer of the ITB, and the anterolateral capsule (**Fig. 1**). Due to the debate on the anterolateral complex and its potential role in rotatory knee stability, the structural properties of the

[a] Orthopaedic Robotics Laboratory, University of Pittsburgh, 300 Technology Drive, Pittsburgh, PA 15219, USA; [b] Department of Bioengineering, University of Pittsburgh, 3700 O'Hara Street, Pittsburgh, PA 15213, USA; [c] Trauma Department, Hannover Medical School (MHH), Carl-Neuberg-Street 1, Hannover 30625, Germany; [d] Department of Orthopaedic Surgery, University of Pittsburgh, 3471 Fifth Avenue, Pittsburgh, PA, USA; [e] UPMC Rooney Sports Complex, Sports Medicine Fellowship, Department of Orthopaedic Surgery, University of Pittsburgh, UPMC Center for Sports Medicine, 3200 South Water Street, Pittsburgh, PA 15203, USA
* Corresponding author. UPMC Rooney Sports Complex, Sports Medicine Fellowship, Department of Orthopaedic Surgery, University of Pittsburgh, UPMC Center for Sports Medicine, 3200 South Water Street, Pittsburgh, PA 15203.
E-mail address: musahlv@upmc.edu

Clin Sports Med 37 (2018) 41–47
http://dx.doi.org/10.1016/j.csm.2017.07.005
0278-5919/18/© 2017 Elsevier Inc. All rights reserved.

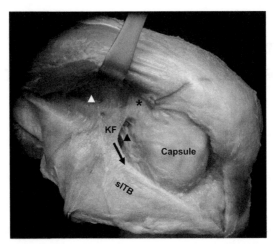

Fig. 1. The anterolateral complex of the knee and its key features. sITB, superficial ITB; KF, Kaplan fibers; *asterisk*, the accessory fiber bundles of the Kaplan fibers that insert on the lateral superior condyle; black triangle, capsulo-osseous layer of the ITB; white triangle, branch of the superior genicular artery; and black arrow, direction of the deep ITB, which merges to the sITB. (*From* Herbst E, Albers M, Burnham JM, et al. The anterolateral complex of the knee: a pictorial essay. Knee Surg Sports Traumatol Arthrosc 2017;25[4]:1011; with permission Springer.)

anterolateral complex as well as its role in providing joint stability have recently been examined.[4–6] For clarification, the term, *anterolateral ligament*, in this article is used as a term describing a thickening of the anterolateral complex, as described by previous research studies.[4–7]

Evidence of the involvement of the anterolateral complex in knee rotatory stability emerged from biomechanical studies, which showed increased rotatory knee instability due to injury of the anterolateral structures in ACL-deficient knees.[1,8–10] The determination of the synergistic roles of the anterolateral complex and the ACL in controlling rotatory knee instability has great clinical implications. Several extra-articular procedures have been developed to supplement ACL reconstruction and improve rotatory knee stability.[11–14] Furthermore, the thorough understanding of the structural properties of the anterolateral complex of the knee would benefit patients with residual rotatory knee instability after ACL reconstruction. Understanding of the structural properties of the anterolateral complex of the knee provides an assessment of how the overall tissue complex behaves, whereas the mechanical properties of the anterolateral complex describe the quality of the tissue itself independent of the geometry. Clinically, the structural properties of grafts used for reconstruction procedures should be comparable to the native tissue.

The aim of this article is to provide a summary on the evidence regarding the structural properties of the anterolateral complex of the knee, its components, and their implications in rotatory knee stability in the clinical setting.

STRUCTURAL PROPERTIES OF THE ANTEROLATERAL COMPLEX

The anterolateral structures of the knee have been the focus of several investigations that characterize the structural properties of the anterolateral complex.[6,7,15] The key structural properties of the anterolateral complex that were investigated are ultimate load (the highest load a tissue can withstand before failure) and stiffness (force

generated per unit deformation). The structural properties of the anterolateral complex provide insight on its relative contribution to joint stability. In addition, the description of a distinct ligament in the anterolateral capsule, the anterolateral ligament, has precipitated much research into its structural properties.[4–7]

Quantitative data on the location and structural properties of the anterolateral ligament have been obtained to guide future anterolateral ligament reconstructions on the appropriate graft selection and placement.[4] To quantify the structural properties of the anterolateral ligament, uniaxial tensile testing of the femur–anterolateral ligament–tibia complex was performed with the femur and tibia secured at 30° of knee flexion. The anterolateral ligament was identified through a combined outside-in and inside-out anatomic dissection with the knee flexed between 30° and 60° and internally rotated. At this position, the taut fibers of the lateral capsule located posterior and proximal to the lateral femoral epicondyle and coursing to the area between Gerdy tubercle and the anterior margin of the fibular head defined the anterolateral ligament. For the anterolateral ligament, the ultimate load was 175 N (95% CI of 139 N–211 N) and stiffness was 20 N/mm (95% CI of 16 N/mm–25 N/mm). The most common mode of failure was a bony avulsion from the tibia (n = 6) followed by failure at the femoral insertion (n = 4), midsubstance (n = 4), and tibial insertion (n = 1). Kennedy and colleagues[4] concluded that most soft tissue grafts would be suitable for extra-articular knee reconstructions because grafts used for extra-articular reconstruction procedures either match or surpass the ultimate loads of the anterolateral ligament.

The structural properties of the anterolateral ligament were further investigated by other investigators to better understand its contribution to knee stability and to determine suitable grafts for reconstruction techniques.[7] The anterolateral ligament was defined as the capsular thickening in the anterolateral region of the knee with the knee flexed and internally rotated. The dissection of the anterolateral ligament was performed starting from the femoral origin to the tibial insertion in the proximal to distal direction. Uniaxial tensile tests were performed on the femur–anterolateral ligament–tibia complex, with the knee fixed in approximately 30° to 40° of flexion. The ultimate load of the anterolateral ligament was found to be 204.8 N ± 115 N and the stiffness was 41.9 N/mm ± 25.7 N/mm. The most common mode of failure was at the midsubstance (n = 10), femoral detachment (n = 2), tibial detachment (n = 1), and a Segond fracture (n = 1). Helito and colleagues[7] concluded that based on the strength (ultimate load) of the anterolateral ligament, simple bands of autologous or homologous grafts may be used for ligament reconstruction.

The structural properties of the anterolateral ligament were also compared with the ITB and gracilis grafts to determine the most appropriate graft for the anterolateral ligament.[5] Grafts of the ITB and gracilis were harvested, whereas the anterolateral ligament remained attached to the femur and tibia. The anterolateral ligament was defined as the fibrous structure having a tibial insertion midway between Gerdy tubercle and the fibular head and a femoral insertion proximal and posterior to the lateral femoral epicondyle. Uniaxial tensile tests of the ITB and gracilis grafts were performed in isolation, whereas the anterolateral ligament was tested in situ with its bony attachments to the femur and tibia. During uniaxial tensile tests of the femur–anterolateral ligament–tibia complex, the femur and tibia were positioned with the knee at full extension. The anterolateral ligament was found to have an ultimate load of 141 N ± 40.6 N, ultimate elongation of 6.2 mm ± 3.2 mm, and a stiffness of 21 N/mm ± 8.2 N/mm. The anterolateral ligament was significantly less stiff than the ITB (39.9 N/mm ± 6.0 N/mm) and gracilis (131.7 N/mm ± 43.7 N/mm) grafts, had significantly lower ultimate load than the gracilis (200.7 N/mm ± 48.7 N), and significantly less ultimate elongation than the ITB (20.8 mm ± 14.7 mm) and gracilis (19.9 mm ± 6.5 mm) grafts.

Wytrykowski and colleagues[5] concluded, however, that the ITB had structural properties that most closely resembled the anterolateral ligament.

To better understand the role of the anterolateral ligament in patients with anterolateral rotational instability, the structural properties of the femur–anterolateral ligament–tibia complex and mechanical properties of the anterolateral ligament were quantified.[6] Using a total of 4 fresh-frozen knees, the anterolateral ligament was identified at 90° of flexion and defined as the ligamentous structure connecting the lateral femoral epicondyle and the anterolateral proximal tibia. The uniaxial tensile tests were performed with the fibers of the anterolateral ligament aligned with the direction of loading. To determine the mechanical properties of the anterolateral ligament, cross-sectional area measurements were made using histologic samples from the anterolateral ligament after uniaxial tensile tests. The specific failure modes for each test specimen were not reported. The anterolateral ligament had an ultimate load of 49.0 N $\pm$ 14.6 N and stiffness of 2.6 N/mm $\pm$ 0.9 N/mm. Ultimate stress was reported to be 32.8 MPa $\pm$ 4.0 MPa and a modulus of 1.2 N/mm^2 $\pm$ 0.4 N/mm^2. The ultimate stress reported for the anterolateral ligament was comparable to true ligaments, such as the ACL (37.8 MPa), medial collateral ligament (MCL) (38.6 MPa), and posterior cruciate ligament (PCL) (35.9 MPa).[16,17] Based on the structural properties of the anterolateral ligament found in this study, the investigators concluded that the anterolateral ligament is not a primary stabilizer of the knee joint due to significantly lower ultimate loads compared with true ligaments found in the knee.

The authors also investigated the role of the anterolateral capsule in knee stability by determining the structural properties of the anterolateral capsule. In addition, the structural properties of the ITB were determined because it is a commonly used graft for extra-articular tenodesis.[18] Dissection of the anterolateral capsule assured that the newly proposed ligament was contained within the construct dissected by sectioning the capsule 2 cm anterior to the lateral collateral ligament (LCL).[19] A discrete thickening of the capsule was found in only 2 of 9 knees. A 15-cm by 1-cm wide strip of the ITB was cut and left attached to Gerdy tubercle. Uniaxial tensile tests for the anterolateral capsule were performed with the knee in 45° of flexion to assure the fibers of the lateral capsule were most evenly loaded. In addition, the tibia with respect to the femur was adjusted for each specimen by 2°$\pm$ 4° of varus/valgus and 0°$\pm$ 1° of internal/external rotation to uniformly load the capsule. The anterolateral capsule showed significantly lower ultimate load (319.7 N $\pm$ 212.6 N vs 487.9 N $\pm$ 156.9 N) and stiffness (26.0 N/mm $\pm$ 11.5 N/mm vs 73.2 N/mm $\pm$ 24.1 N/mm) as well as significantly higher ultimate elongation (15.5 mm $\pm$ 7.3 mm vs 8.6 mm $\pm$ 1.4 mm) than the ITB. The most common failure mode for the capsule was in the midsubstance (n = 3) and tibial insertion site (n = 3). The remaining 2 specimens failed at the femoral insertion site. The structural properties of the anterolateral capsule were significantly lower compared with the ITB, and therefore extra-articular reconstruction using an ITB graft may result in overconstraint of the ACL-reconstructed knee.

Based on the results of these studies, the anterolateral ligament has a lower ultimate load and stiffness compared with true tendons and ligaments in the knee (**Tables 1 and 2**). For example, the stiffness of the anterolateral ligament is approximately 21.5 N/mm, which is 91% lower than the ACL and approximately 78% lower than the ITB. All major ligamentous structures of the knee (ACL, MCL, PCL, and LCL) were at least 3 times stiffer than values determined for the anterolateral ligament. The ultimate load of the anterolateral ligament is approximately 143 N, more than 69% weaker than the LCL. Compared with the ACL, the anterolateral ligament is more than 93% weaker.

Table 1
Structural properties of defined structures of the knee

Structure	Stiffness (N/MM)	Ultimate Load (N)
ACL[20]	242 ± 28	2160 ± 157
MCL[21]	63 ± 14	799 ± 209
LCL[22]	82 ± 25	460 ± 163
PCL[23]	204 ± 49	1627 ± 491
ITB[24]	97 ± 35	582 ± 193

DISCUSSION

Based on the studies that investigated the structural properties of the anterolateral complex of the knee, it was evident that the entire anterolateral complex plays a minimal role in providing stability at the knee joint. Furthermore, although previous studies have reported the presence of a ligament in this region of the knee, the structural properties of the anterolateral ligament were found much lower than true ligaments of the knee (see **Table 1**).[17,20,25] Differences in the structural properties of the anterolateral ligament reported by several studies[4–7] may be due to differences in the test setup, especially alignment of fibers due to knee flexion. Furthermore, the definition of the anterolateral ligament and tissue included in the complex based on dissection was different between studies and could have significantly altered the geometry-dependent structural properties of the anterolateral ligament.

Additionally, the mechanical properties of the anterolateral ligament reported by 1 study showed comparable ultimate stress values to true ligaments in the knee.[6] This, however, may be due to the underestimation of the cross-sectional area measurements used to calculate stress because they were taken after the ligaments failed during the load-to-failure testing. The different modes of failure reported during the uniaxial tensile tests of the anterolateral ligament suggest the structure does not behave like a ligament and is much weaker. When considering that failure occurs at the weakest point of the bone-tissue-bone complex, it seems that the multiple failure locations reported by all studies may be due to lack of inherent organization of the capsular tissue in 1 direction. Thus, future studies should investigate the structural properties of the anterolateral complex using a biaxial test setup to determine if the anterolateral complex transmits loads in multiple directions. Overall, the results from these studies show no evidence that a ligament exists in the anterolateral region of the knee; rather, the anterolateral capsule acts more like a sheet of tissue.

Table 2
Structural properties of the proposed ligamentous structure (anterolateral ligament)

Anterolateral Ligament Studies	Anterolateral Ligament Stiffness (N/MM)	Anterolateral Ligament Ultimate Load (N)
Helito et al,[7] 2016	42 ± 26	205 ± 115
Kennedy et al,[4] 2015	20 ± 8	175 ± 65
Wytrykowski et al,[5] 2016	21 ± 8	141 ± 41
Zens et al,[6] 2015	3 ± 1	50 ± 15

CLINICAL IMPLICATIONS

The structural properties of the anterolateral structures of the knee suggest that both the anterolateral capsule and the anterolateral ligament exhibit lower ultimate load and stiffness than true ligaments of the knee.[17,20,25] Although these results provide objective insight to treating physicians, more research is needed to explore surgical indications for anterolateral soft tissue reconstruction. There is a risk of over-constraining the knee with procedures, such as the extra-articular tenodesis of the anterolateral complex of the knee, which provides a nonanatomic reconstruction of the anterolateral complex, because most grafts used have a much higher stiffness than the capsule.[2,13,26] Some investigators advocate the addition of the extra-articular tenodesis of the anterolateral structures in ACL-deficient knee with marked rotational instability and revision cases.[27]

SUMMARY

The entire anterolateral complex has an impact on rotatory and translational stability of the knee. Reconstruction methods need to be adapted on the pattern of injury and the amount of rotatory knee instability. Although the surgical indications to perform soft tissue reconstruction of the anterolateral structure of the knee have not been thoroughly vetted, additional mechanical studies are needed to support these clinical decisions. Further biomechanical analysis of the anterolateral complex would potentially help physicians to determine precise surgical indication for individualized surgical treatment, and improve patient surgical outcomes. Specifically, biaxial testing of the anterolateral complex should be conducted to determine if the anterolateral complex transmits loads in multiple directions.

REFERENCES

1. Kittl C, El-Daou H, Athwal KK, et al. The role of the anterolateral structures and the ACL in controlling laxity of the intact and ACL-deficient knee. Am J Sports Med 2016;44(2):345–54.
2. Araujo PH, Kfuri Junior M, Ohashi B, et al. Individualized ACL reconstruction. Knee Surg Sports Traumatol Arthrosc 2014;22(9):1966–75.
3. Inderhaug E, Stephen JM, Williams A, et al. Biomechanical comparison of anterolateral procedures combined with anterior cruciate ligament reconstruction. Am J Sports Med 2017;45(2):347–54.
4. Kennedy MI, Claes S, Fuso FA, et al. The anterolateral ligament: an anatomic, radiographic, and biomechanical analysis. Am J Sports Med 2015;43(7): 1606–15.
5. Wytrykowski K, Swider P, Reina N, et al. Cadaveric study comparing the biomechanical properties of grafts used for knee anterolateral ligament reconstruction. Arthroscopy 2016;32(11):2288–94.
6. Zens M, Feucht MJ, Ruhhammer J, et al. Mechanical tensile properties of the anterolateral ligament. J Exp Orthop 2015;2(1):7.
7. Helito CP, Bonadio MB, Rozas JS, et al. Biomechanical study of strength and stiffness of the knee anterolateral ligament. BMC Musculoskelet Disord 2016;17:193.
8. Suero EM, Njoku IU, Voigt MR, et al. The role of the iliotibial band during the pivot shift test. Knee Surg Sports Traumatol Arthrosc 2013;21(9):2096–100.
9. Monaco E, Ferretti A, Labianca L, et al. Navigated knee kinematics after cutting of the ACL and its secondary restraint. Knee Surg Sports Traumatol Arthrosc 2012; 20(5):870–7.

10. Yamamoto Y, Hsu WH, Fisk JA, et al. Effect of the iliotibial band on knee biomechanics during a simulated pivot shift test. J Orthop Res 2006;24(5):967–73.

11. Samuelson M, Draganich LF, Zhou X, et al. The effects of knee reconstruction on combined anterior cruciate ligament and anterolateral capsular deficiencies. Am J Sports Med 1996;24(4):492–7.

12. Chahla J, Menge TJ, Mitchell JJ, et al. Anterolateral ligament reconstruction technique: an anatomic-based approach. Arthrosc Tech 2016;5(3):e453–7.

13. Marcacci M, Zaffagnini S, Iacono F, et al. Arthroscopic intra- and extra-articular anterior cruciate ligament reconstruction with gracilis and semitendinosus tendons. Knee Surg Sports Traumatol Arthrosc 1998;6(2):68–75.

14. Noyes FR, Huser LE, Jurgensmeier D, et al. Is an anterolateral ligament reconstruction required in ACL-reconstructed knees with associated injury to the anterolateral structures? A robotic analysis of rotational knee stability. Am J Sports Med 2017;45(5):1018–27.

15. Thein R, Boorman-Padgett J, Stone K, et al. Biomechanical assessment of the anterolateral ligament of the knee: a secondary restraint in simulated tests of the pivot shift and of anterior stability. J Bone Joint Surg Am 2016;98(11):937–43.

16. Quapp KM, Weiss JA. Material characterization of human medial collateral ligament. J Biomech Eng 1998;120(6):757–63.

17. Noyes FR, Butler DL, Grood ES, et al. Biomechanical analysis of human ligament grafts used in knee-ligament repairs and reconstructions. J Bone Joint Surg Am 1984;66(3):344–52.

18. Rahnemai-Azar AA, Miller RM, Guenther D, et al. Structural properties of the anterolateral capsule and iliotibial band of the knee. Am J Sports Med 2016;44(4):892–7.

19. Claes S, Vereecke E, Maes M, et al. Anatomy of the anterolateral ligament of the knee. J Anat 2013;223(4):321–8.

20. Woo SL, Hollis JM, Adams DJ, et al. Tensile properties of the human femur-anterior cruciate ligament-tibia complex. The effects of specimen age and orientation. Am J Sports Med 1991;19(3):217–25.

21. Wilson WT, Deakin AH, Payne AP, et al. Comparative analysis of the structural properties of the collateral ligaments of the human knee. J Orthop Sports Phys Ther 2012;42(4):345–51.

22. Ciccone WJ II, Bratton DR, Weinstein DM, et al. Structural properties of lateral collateral ligament reconstruction at the fibular head. Am J Sports Med 2006;34(1):24–8.

23. Prietto MP, Bain JR, Stonebrook SN, et al. Tensile strength of the human posterior cruciate ligament (PCL). Trans Orthop Res Soc 1988;13:195.

24. Merican AM, Sanghavi S, Iranpour F, et al. The structural properties of the lateral retinaculum and capsular complex of the knee. J Biomech 2009;42(14):2323–9.

25. Race A, Amis AA. The mechanical properties of the two bundles of the human posterior cruciate ligament. J Biomech 1994;27(1):13–24.

26. Schon JM, Moatshe G, Brady AW, et al. Anatomic anterolateral ligament reconstruction of the knee leads to overconstraint at any fixation angle. Am J Sports Med 2016;44(10):2546–56.

27. Bonasia DE, D'Amelio A, Pellegrino P, et al. Anterolateral ligament of the knee: back to the future in anterior cruciate ligament reconstruction. Orthop Rev 2015;7(2):5773.

Secondary Stabilizers of Tibial Rotation in the Intact and Anterior Cruciate Ligament Deficient Knee

Daniel James Kaplan, BA*, Laith M. Jazrawi, MD

KEYWORDS

- Anterior cruciate ligament • Iliotibial band • Anterolateral capsule • Lateral meniscus
- Anterolateral ligament

KEY POINTS

- The anterior cruciate ligament is the primary stabilizer to tibial rotation.
- The iliotibial band is the main secondary stabilizer to tibial rotation, particularly at higher flexion angles at which the anterior cruciate ligament plays less of a role.
- The anterolateral complex is an important stabilizer for tibial rotation, but its exact anatomic definition remains ambiguous, as does its biomechanical function.
- The lateral meniscus also functions as a secondary stabilizer of tibial rotation.

INTRODUCTION

The controversy regarding the existence and possible function of the anterolateral ligament (ALL) has reinvigorated interest in rotational control of the knee joint. This is particularly true of internal rotation (IR), and anterolateral rotary instability. With anterior cruciate ligament (ACL) reconstruction failure rates ranging from 0% to 14%, many in the sports medicine community are pointing toward compromised anterolateral restraints as the underlying culprit.[1,2] The anterolateral complex includes the iliotibial band (ITB), the anterolateral capsule (ALC), lateral meniscus (LM), and lateral collateral ligament (LCL). This article provides breakdown of these structures, their functions, biomechanical properties, and clinical importance, based on a thorough review of available literature.

WHAT IS THE PRIMARY STABILIZER OF TIBIAL ROTATION?

The primary stabilizer of tibial rotation must first be defined before any secondary stabilizers can be named. In 1980, Butler and colleagues,[3] introduced the concept of the

Disclosure: The authors have no relevant disclosures.
Department of Orthopaedic Surgery, New York University Langone Medical Center, 301 East 17th Street, New York, NY 10010, USA
* Corresponding author.
E-mail address: danieljameskaplan@gmail.com

primary restraint. Primary restraint was conceptually explained by Andersen and Dyhre-Poulsen[4] as follows, "cutting a primary restraint results in an increase in joint motion, whereas cutting a secondary restraint will result in an increase of joint motion only in the absence of the primary restraint." This notion was used as the foundation for future biomechanical studies looking to establish the significance of various restraints.

Early research posited the ACL as the primary restraint to tibial IR—particularly at low flexion angles. In 1981, Lipke and colleagues[5] found that isolated transection of the ACL resulted in significantly increased tibial IR, which increased even more so with subsequent sectioning of the ALC and LCL. Transection the lateral structures first and leaving the ACL intact, however, resulted in no significant difference to internal rotation. Also using cadaveric specimens, one study testing the biomechanical properties of intra-articular and extra-articular ACL reconstructions and a second study investigating the efficacy of a pivot shift testing mechanism[6] both found cutting the ACL alone led to significantly increased internal rotation—although the latter group did not find this to be true at 90° of knee flexion.[6,7] Several studies that examined the differences and importance of the 2 bundles of the ACL, confirm the previous findings that isolated transection of the ACL results in significantly increased IR of the tibia.[8–10] Biomechanically, tibial torque is believed to cause winding of the ACL fibers around each other, which results in loading of the ligament and resistance to rotation.[9]

An increasing body of evidence, however, suggests that the ACL is not, in fact, critical for IR stability. Andersen and Dyhre-Poulsen,[4] in a study of cadaver knees found that at the time of transection of the ACL, IR increased significantly when compared with normal knees at 10° and 30° of flexion, but not at 50°, 70°, or 90°. The group concluded the ACL was a primary stabilizer at low flexion angles. A classic study by Lane and colleagues,[11] found transection of the ACL did not result in any significant increase in IR; however, with only 14 cadaver specimens, this study may have been underpowered. Kittl and colleagues,[12] compared the percentage contribution to IR resistance of the ACL and several anterolateral structures and found the ACL was the chief restraint to IR only at full extension. Similarly, Kanamori and colleagues,[13] found no significant differences between ACL-intact and ACL-deficient knees, reporting a less than 3° difference between groups at all flexion angles during isolated tibial loading and during a simulated pivot shift test. At 15° of flexion, Oh and colleagues,[14] found transection of the ACL led to a significant, but small (.7°) change compared with intact knees. Several other studies found slightly larger degree differences between ACL-intact and ACL-deficient knees in response to IR. However, because of sample sizes and type of statistical testing, these still relatively minor IR increases were not found to be significant.[15–20] The ACL is likely the primary stabilizer of tibial internal rotation, particularly from 0° to 30° of flexion. At flexion angles greater than 30°, the ACL is still likely the chief restraint to internal tibial rotation, but the contribution of the anterolateral complex increases with increased flexion.

SECONDARY STABILIZERS
Iliotibial Band

The importance of the ITB was first elucidated by Kaplan[21] in 1958. He defined the ITB as a stabilizing ligament attached to the lateral femoral condyle at a fixed point and attached to Gerdy tubercle where it moves forward in extension and backward in flexion.[21] The ITB is a thickening of deep fascia, intimately connected with the tensor fasciae latae anteriorly and gluteus maximus posteriorly. It extends laterally from the iliac crest to the tibia, with connecting fibers to the femur along its length.[21] At the knee joint, the superficial layer begins to branch obliquely in an anterolateral direction, covering the patella, patellar tendon, and Gerdy's tubercle.[22] The deep portion of the ITB also contains a distinct set of fibers that run from their origin at the lateral femoral supraepicondylar region to their insertion on the proximal tibia between the fibular head and Gerdy's tubercle. These fibers are often referred to as the *Kaplan fibers* and are believed to be particularly important in the role of ITB as a secondary stabilizer to tibial internal rotation.[21,23]

Given its extra-articular and anterolateral location, the ITB has a much longer lever arm than the ACL when resisting IR. Despite this perceived anatomic advantage, the ITB in the setting of an intact ACL does not play a major role. Huser and colleagues,[24] used 19 fresh-frozen cadavers to determine the role of the ITB and ACL in intact knees. Sectioning the ITB alone led to a significant increase in tibial IR of 3.0° at 60° and 2.2° at 90° of knee flexion. Consistent with previous studies, sectioning the ITB made the least difference at 25° of knee flexion (0.4° increase; **Table 1**). Although these increases were statistically significant, the authors concluded they were likely clinically insignificant.[24]

A recent 2016 study found the ITB to be the single most important contributor to internal rotation resistance, even in the intact knee.[12] The authors found the ACL was the only significant contributor of IR resistance at full extension. At 30°, 60°, and 90° of flexion, the superficial ITB and the deep ITB (Kaplan fibers included) both contributed significant resistance to tibial IR, with the superficial ITB contributing more resistance at higher flexion angles, and the deep ITB resisting most of the load at lower flexion angles (30°). The ITB as a whole was found to provide 44%, 76%, and 71% of IR torque resistance at 30°, 60°, and 90° of knee flexion, respectively.[12] Sonnery-Cottet and colleagues,[25] in a 2016 study, also investigated the role of ALL and ITB in ACL intact and deficient cadaver specimens. Isolated transection of the ITB in an otherwise intact knee resulted in a significant increase in IR (21.9% additional IR) at low flexion (20°), whereas transection of the ACL had a larger effect at 90° of knee flexion. With the ACL and ALL sectioned, they again found the ITB to resist IR torque more at lower flexion angles. Additional transection of the ITB induced a further significant increase in IR of 42.3% at 20° and 37.7% at 90°.

This evidence suggests the ITB is likely the most important secondary stabilizer of tibial IR, particularly at higher flexion angles. Clinically this was shown in a study by Terry and colleagues,[26] that evaluated 80 patients with ACL tears, of which 76 had concomitant injury to the ITB. The severity of the ITB injury (particularly the deep ITB) in ACL-deficient patients correlated significantly with abnormal motion detected on physical examination determined by the pivot shift grade, Lachman test, and lateral joint line opening at 30°. The status of the ITB thus should be considered when evaluating an ACL injury particularly in the chronic setting with a high pivot-shift grade or a failed previous reconstruction.

Anterolateral Capsule

Recent interest in the ALC has challenged the importance of the ITB, with some investigators suggesting the ALC may in fact be the paramount secondary stabilizer.[27–29] Some experts suggest a lateral extra-articular tenodesis (or ALL reconstruction) should be performed in select cases, whereas others argue these procedures potentially overconstrain the knee.[28,30–32] At the heart of this controversy is the debate over the clinical relevance and anatomic properties of the capsule, namely, whether it should be considered a true ligament or only a potential thickening.[33–38] Claes and colleagues,[37] are credited with popularizing the current concept of the anterolateral ligament and described it as, "a distinct ligamentous structure clearly distinguishable

Table 1
Key studies examining the role of the iliotibial band in the knee

Reference Information			Methods	Main Findings	
Lead Author, Year	Journal	6DFR	Force Used	ACL Intact	ACL Deficient
Wroble et al,[48] 1993	AJSM	Yes	5 Nm IR, 0°, 30°, 60°, and 90°		IR↑ SS/CS >30° of kf°
Terry et al,[26] 1993	AJSM	Live patients	Injury correlated with abnormal motion		ITB injury highly correlated to abnormal motion grade
Huser et al,[24] 2016	Arthroscopy	Yes	5 Nm IR, 25°, 60°, and 90°	IR↑ Conc: *SS, not CS*	
Kittl et al,[12] 2016	AJSM	Yes	5 Nm IR, 0°, 30°, 60°, and 90°	Both sITT and dcITT had IR ↑ SS, CS at 30°, 60°, and 90° -sITT > important at high kf° -dcITT: > important at low kf°	dcITT SS/CS at 0° Both sITT and dcITT SS/CS at 30°, 60° and 90°
Sonnery-Cottet et al,[25] 2016	AJSM	No	2 Nm 20°, 90°	IR↑ SS/CS at 20°, not at 90°	IR↑ SS/CS at 20°, not at 90°

Main findings: Results after transecting the ITB in study of interest.
Abbreviations: 6DFR, 6 degree of freedom robot; AJSM, American Journal of Sports Medicine; CS, clinically significant (as determined by authors of individual papers); dcITT, deep ITB; kf°, knee flexion angles; sITT, superficial ITB; SS, statistically significant ($P<.05$).

from the anterolateral joint capsule, originating at the prominence of the lateral femoral epicondyle, slightly anterior to the origin of the LCL, and coursing obliquely to the anterolateral aspect of the proximal tibia." They determined that this layer was discretely separate from the deep layer (Kaplan fibers) of the ITB, which they found to only go as distal as the lateral epicondyle, not the tibia. Based on the author's own work, however,[39] the ALC does not seem to be a distinct ligament. For the purposes of this review, the anterolateral capsule will, therefore, be defined as a discrete mid-third anterolateral capsular thickening of approximately 2 to 4 mm coursing from the lateral epicondyle to the tibia midway between Gerdy's tubercle and the fibular head (**Fig. 1**A, B).[33,35]

The biomechanical properties of the ALC have been extensively studied to better understand its significance. Rahnemai-Azar and colleagues,[35] used 9 intact cadaveric knee specimens to examine the differences between the 2 structures in the physiologic setting. When compared with the ITB, the ALC had significantly lower ultimate load (319.7 N vs 487.9 N) and ultimate stiffness (26.0 N/mm vs 73.2 N/mm). The ALC also elongated nearly twice as much (15.5 mm vs 8.6 mm) under strain. These considerably weaker structural properties suggest the ALC is not as clinically important as the ITB, which is theorized to play the same role in anterolateral restraint (**Table 2**).

Because the ALC is likely a secondary stabilizer, it is not surprising that studies examining its role only in ACL-intact knees do not find it to have a significant role in preventing tibial IR. With an intact ACL, sectioning the entire ALC as posterior as the LCL resulted in no change in IR or external rotation, suggesting it had no role in IR resistance.[5] A biomechanical study using 19 fresh-frozen ACL-intact cadaver knees transected either the ALC then the ITB, or the ITB followed by the ALC to examine their ability to resist IR. With solely the ALC sectioned, IR increased nonsignificantly by less than 2° at each flexion angle tested (25°, 60°, and 90°). It was only when the ITB was sectioned in addition to the ALC that IR significantly increased. The authors concluded the ALC could not be considered a primary stabilizer of tibial IR and only would affect IR if the ITB was also injured. Even in this case, the authors felt this would be clinically detectable.[24]

Most studies that examined the role of the ALC in the ACL-deficient knee also found that it did not play a major role in restricting tibial IR. Spencer and colleagues,[1]

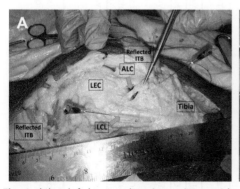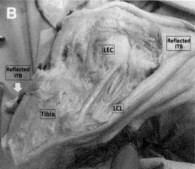

Fig. 1. (*A*) A left knee cadaveric specimen without an easily identifiable ALC. The ITB has been reflected to better see the underlying anatomy. LEC, lateral epicondyle. (*B*) A right knee cadaveric specimen with an isolated ALC. Again, the ITB has been reflected to better see the underlying anatomy.

Table 2
Key studies examining the role of the anterolateral capsule in the knee

Reference Information		Methods		Main Findings	
Lead Author, Year	Journal	6DFR	Force Used	ACL Intact	ACL Deficient
Monaco et al,[16] 2010	Orthopedics	No	Max manually possible 0°, 15°, 30°, 45°, 60°, 90°		IR ↑ 0°–60° SS at 0° only
Parsons et al,[20] 2015	AJSM	Yes	5 Nm IR 0°, 15°, 25°, 35°, 45°, 60°, 75°, and 90°	IR↑ at all kf°, and ALC > ACL >30°	
Rasmussen et al,[29] 2016	AJSM	Yes	5 Nm IR 0°, 15°, 30°, 45°, 60°, 90°		IR↑ (avg 2.7°) at all kf°, largest at 60° SS and CS
Spencer et al,[1] 2015	AJSM	No	Manual pivot shift 5-Nm internal rotation moment and a 10-Nm valgus force 0°		IR↑ SS compared with intact knee, but no difference with ACL sectioned knee
Huser et al,[24] 2016	Arthroscopy	Yes	5 Nm IR	IR ↑ <0.5° at all kf° Conclusion: Not SS or CS	
Kittl et al,[12] 2016	AJSM	Yes	5 Nm IR, 0°, 30°, 60°, and 90°	Not SS or CS at any kf°	Not SS or CS at any kf°
Sonnery-Cottet et al,[25] 2016	AJSM	No	2 Nm 20°, 90°	IR ↑ SS/CS at 20°, 90°	IR ↑ SS/CS at 20°, 90°
Rahnemai-Azar et al,[35] 2016	AJSM	yes	Load to failure, elongation, stiffness	ALC significantly less than load to failure, and stiffness than ITB; ALC significantly greater than elongation than ITB	
Guenther et al,[36] 2017	AJSM	Yes	7-Nm IR 30°, 60°, 90°	ALC experienced SS less than force than other structures at all kf°	ALC experienced SS less than force than other structures at all kf°

Abbreviations: 6DFR, 6 degree of freedom robot; AJSM, American Journal of Sports Medicine; CS, clinically significant (as determined by authors of individual papers); kf°, knee flexion angles; SS, statistically significant (P<.05).

measured the IR of the tibia after transection of the ACL in 12 fresh-frozen cadaver knees and found sectioning the ALC only increased IR by 2°. They found this increase to be statistically significant but believed the magnitude was of little clinical importance. Unlike most biomechanical studies discussed in this review, this study did not use a 6-degrees-of-freedom robot to apply force moments, rather, a human-applied force manually.[1]

Kittl and colleagues,[12] defined the ALL as the remaining fibers after removal of the deep ITB (which included the Kaplan fibers), and the ALC was defined as the midthird lateral capsular ligament. In the ACL-intact specimens, they found the ALC did not significantly contribute to IR resistance at any flexion angle tested, only contributing between .7% and 4.1%. When the ACL was transected, the ALC resistance to IR did not significantly increase. A unique study by Guenther and colleagues,[36] measured the force transmitted by the ALC in its longitudinal direction and the force transmitted between the capsular regions. It was determined that in the ACL-intact and ACL-deficient knees, the ALC transmitted negligible forces longitudinally (which represents its ability to resist IR), indicating the ALC does not function as a traditional ligament (which does resist forces parallel to its longitudinal axis). Conversely, The ALC transmitted a significant load perpendicular to its longitudinal axis, particularly in the ACL-deficient knee, which is typical of a sheet of tissue. These authors concluded the ALC may be important for its role in IR restraint but as a total capsular structure rather than a discrete ligament.

The nondistinct nature of the ALC has resulted in different characterizations of the ALL. As a result, studies have defined the ALL differently in their methods, and their dissection techniques also vary considerably. Monaco and colleagues[16] dissected 6 ACL-deficient hip-to-toe fresh-frozen cadaver specimens. Sectioning off what they termed, the *anterolateral femorotibial ligament*, resulted in significantly increased IR between 0° and 60°.This investigation, however, was performed before many of the anatomic studies previously mentioned. The authors made a 2-cm-long incision through the anterolateral femorotibial ligament but fail to describe what portion of the ALC or ITB they transected. Parsons and colleagues,[20] evaluated the role of the ACL, LCL, and ALC in 12 fresh-frozen cadaver specimens. Because of the randomized nature of their sequential sectioning, they did not directly compare the contribution of the ALC in ACL-intact versus ACL-deficient knees, instead relying on the principle of superimposition. Similar to other studies, the ALC contributed more to the IR moment greater than 30° of knee flexion, whereas the ACL played a larger role at nearly full extension. The authors removed the superficial ITB but left the deep ITB as part of the ALC they were testing. As has been shown, the deep ITB (including Kaplan fibers) plays a major role in IR control. It is therefore difficult to draw meaningful conclusions from their results.

Several recent studies investigated the role of the ALC with clearly defined dissection protocols and found it played a significant role in resisting tibial IR. Rasmussen and colleagues,[29] found sectioning of the ALC in ACL-deficient knees resulted in 2.7° of additional IR in response to 5-N-m in 10 fresh-frozen cadaveric specimens. Another dissection study evaluated the ALC in knees with either the ACL intact and ITB transected or with only the ACL transected. In the ACL-deficient knees, additional transection of the ALC resulted in significantly increased IR at both 20° and 90° (only degrees tested). Similarly, in knees with an intact ACL, but transected ITB, additional sectioning of the ALC resulted in significantly increased IR at both 20° and 90°.[25] Both groups concluded the ALC was important for rotational control of the knee.

It is difficult to make any definitive statements regarding the ALC at this time. As Roessler and colleagues note,[40] because the structure is not discrete, different authors may be describing completely different tissues. Furthermore, the description of the structure varies based on if the cadaver specimens, like most in this review, were fresh-frozen or embalmed as in the work by Claes and colleagues.[36] Many studies also seem to be including the deep ITB with the ALC, further complicating matters. It is likely the capsular thickening plays a role in rotational stability but likely a much less important one than the ITB.

Lateral Meniscus

The function of the menisci is to decrease tibiofemoral contact stresses and to facilitate normal joint kinematics. Unlike the medial meniscus, which has a role as an important secondary stabilizer to anterior translation, lateral meniscectomy is found to result in minimal additional translation.[41] It is theorized that this discrepancy is caused by the LM's lack of significant posterior wedge effect and less firm capsular attachments to the tibial plateau.[42] The LM, however, has been found to be an important secondary restraint to tibial IR.

The role of the LM in resisting IR during a mechanized pivot was investigated using 10 fresh-frozen cadaveric hip-to-toe specimen pairs. In response to a combined axial and rotary load, lateral meniscectomy after ACL transection resulted in significantly increased additional anterior translation of the lateral knee compartment, signifying internal rotation. Subsequent removal of the medial meniscus had no effect. Conversely, in ACL-deficient knees with the medial meniscus already removed, subsequent removal of the LM resulted in significantly increased anterior translation of the lateral compartment.[43] Similar results were found when evaluating the effect of lateral meniscal root tears on stability in 8 fresh-frozen ACL-deficient cadaveric knees.[44]

Clinical studies have paralleled biomechanical studies. Hosseini and colleagues,[45] evaluated 21 patients with either isolated ACL injury, ACL injury with concomitant LM injury, or ACL injury with concomitant medial meniscus injury. Knee kinematics during stair climbing were compared between the injured and healthy contralateral knee using dual fluoroscopic imaging. Although no differences were found to be significant, the ACL-deficient group with concomitant LM injury had a mean additional 3.0° of IR when compared with the normal contralateral knee. Musahl and colleagues,[46] found similar results during evaluation of 41 patients with confirmed ACL injuries. The presence or absence of concomitant injuries was determined by 2 blinded radiologists, and a standardized (blinded clinician-applied) pivot shift was then performed under anesthesia. The amount of tibial rotation was quantified using previously validated video analysis techniques. Injury to the LM resulted in significantly more anterior translation of the lateral compartment in response to a combined axial and rotary load.

Both biomechanical and clinical studies support the role of the LM as an important secondary stabilizer to tibial IR. However, unlike the ITB and ALC, the meniscus is not designed to resist force.[47] Similarly, because the meniscus does provide some resistance, repairing it in patients with ACL injuries may reduce excess force experienced by the graft.

Lateral Collateral Ligament

The LCL originates on the lateral femoral epicondyle posterior and proximal to the insertion of the popliteus and inserts on the anterolateral fibular head. The LCL's primary function is to resist varus stress.[48] Possibly because of this role, there few studies examining the LCL's role in resisting tibial IR. Parsons and colleagues,[20] in a cadaveric study, found the LCL contributed less than 5% of IR resistance at all flexion angles. Conversely, in 10 ACL-deficient cadaveric knees, Zantop and colleagues,[49] found sectioning of the LCL resulted in significantly increased IR at 0°, 30°, and 60° of flexion when a rotatory load of 10 Nm valgus and 4 Nm internal tibial torque were applied. Because of its relative longitudinal course across the knee joint, the LCL is likely unable to act as a major secondary stabilizer of tibial internal rotation.

SUMMARY

Anterolateral rotational instability is a multifactorial phenomenon. Although the ACL is the primary restraint to internal rotation of the tibia, the iliotibial band plays a major role as a secondary stabilizer, particularly at higher flexion angles. Furthermore, thickening of the anterolateral capsular also contributes to tibial internal rotation resistance, but less so than the ITB. The LM also plays a role in resisting tibial internal rotation, which becomes more pronounced in the ACL-deficient knee. Collectively, these tissues form the anterolateral complex and work synergistically as a functional unit to provide rotatory knee stability.[50]

REFERENCES

1. Spencer L, Burkhart TA, Tran MN, et al. Biomechanical analysis of simulated clinical testing and reconstruction of the anterolateral ligament of the knee. Am J Sports Med 2015;43(9):2189–97.
2. Tanaka M, Vyas D, Moloney G, et al. What does it take to have a high-grade pivot shift? Knee Surg Sports Traumatol Arthrosc 2012;20(4):737–42.
3. Butler D, Noyes FR, Grood E. Ligamentous restraints to anterior-posterior drawer in the human knee. A biomechanical study. J Bone Joint Surg Am 1980;62: 259–70.
4. Andersen HN, Dyhre-Poulsen P. The anterior cruciate ligament does play a role in controlling axial rotation in the knee. Knee 1997;5(3):145–9.
5. Lipke J, Janecki C, Nelson C, et al. The role of incompetence of the anterior cruciate and lateral ligaments in anterolateral. J Bone Joint Surg Am 1981;63(6): 954–60.
6. Engebretsen L, Wijdicks CA, Anderson CJ, et al. Evaluation of a simulated pivot shift test: a biomechanical study. Knee Surg Sports Traumatol Arthrosc 2012; 20(4):698–702.
7. Amis AA, Scammell BE. Biomechanics of intra-articular and extra-articular reconstruction of the anterior cruciate ligament. J Bone Joint Surg Br 1993;75(5):812–7.
8. Harms SP, Noyes FR, Grood ES, et al. Anatomic single-graft anterior cruciate ligament reconstruction restores rotational stability: a robotic study in cadaveric knees. Arthroscopy 2015;31(10):1981–90.
9. Markolf KL, Park S, Jackson SR, et al. Anterior-posterior and rotatory stability of single and double-bundle anterior cruciate ligament reconstructions. J Bone Joint Surg Am 2009;91(1):107–18.
10. Lorbach O, Pape D, Maas S, et al. Influence of the anteromedial and posterolateral bundles of the anterior cruciate ligament on external and internal tibiofemoral rotation. Am J Sports Med 2010;38(4):721–7.
11. Lane JG, Irby SE, Kaufman K, et al. The anterior cruciate ligament in controlling axial rotation. An evaluation of its effect. Am J Sports Med 1994;22(2):289–93.
12. Kittl C, El-Daou H, Athwal KK, et al. The role of the anterolateral structures and the ACL in controlling laxity of the intact and ACL-deficient knee. Am J Sports Med 2016;44(2):345–54.

13. Kanamori A, Woo SLY, Ma CB, et al. The forces in the anterior cruciate ligament and knee kinematics during a simulated pivot shift test: a human cadaveric study using robotic technology. Arthroscopy 2000;16(6):633–9.
14. Oh YK, Kreinbrink JL, Ashton-Miller JA, et al. Effect of ACL transection on internal tibial rotation in an in vitro simulated pivot landing. J Bone Joint Surg Am 2011; 93(4):372–80.
15. Diermann N, Schumacher T, Schanz S, et al. Rotational instability of the knee: Internal tibial rotation under a simulated pivot shift test. Arch Orthop Trauma Surg 2009;129(3):353–8.
16. Monaco E, Maestri B, Labianca L, et al. Navigated knee kinematics after tear of the ACL and its secondary restraints: preliminary results. Orthopedics 2010; 33(10 Suppl):87–93.
17. Wünschel M, Müller O, Lo J, et al. The anterior cruciate ligament provides resistance to externally applied anterior tibial force but not to internal rotational torque during simulated weight-bearing flexion. Arthroscopy 2010;26(11):1520–7.
18. Amis AA, Bull AMJ, Lie DTT. Biomechanics of rotational instability and anatomic anterior cruciate ligament reconstruction. Oper Tech Orthop 2005;15(1):29–35.
19. Amis AA. The functions of the fibre bundles of the anterior cruciate ligament in anterior drawer, rotational laxity and the pivot shift. Knee Surg Sports Traumatol Arthrosc 2012;20(4):613–20.
20. Parsons EM, Gee AO, Spiekerman C, et al. The biomechanical function of the anterolateral ligament of the knee. Am J Sports Med 2015;43(3):669–74.
21. Kaplan EB. The iliotibial tract: clinical and morphological significance. J Bone Joint Surg Am 1958;40(1):817–32.
22. Cruells Vieira EL, Vieira EÁ, Teixeira da Silva R, et al. An anatomic study of the iliotibial tract. Arthroscopy 2007;23(3):269–74.
23. Terry G, Hughston J, Norwood L. The anatomy of the iliopatellar band and iliotibial tract. Am J Sports Med 1986;14(1):39–45.
24. Huser LE, Noyes FR, Jurgensmeier D, et al. Anterolateral ligament and iliotibial band control of rotational stability in the anterior cruciate ligament–intact knee: defined by tibiofemoral compartment translations and rotations. Arthroscopy 2016;1–10. http://dx.doi.org/10.1016/j.arthro.2016.08.034.
25. Sonnery-Cottet B, Lutz C, Daggett M, et al. The involvement of the anterolateral ligament in rotational control of the knee. Am J Sports Med 2016;44(5):1209–14.
26. Terry G, Norwood L, Hughston J, et al. How iliotibial tract injuries of the knee combine with acute anterior cruciate ligament tears to influence abnormal anterior tibial displacement. Am J Sports Med 1993;21(1):55–60.
27. Tavlo M, Eljaja S, Jensen JT, et al. The role of the anterolateral ligament in ACL insufficient and reconstructed knees on rotatory stability: a biomechanical study on human cadavers. Scand J Med Sci Sports 2016;26(8):960–6.
28. Nitri M, Rasmussen MT, Williams BT, et al. An in vitro robotic assessment of the anterolateral ligament, part 2 anterolateral ligament reconstruction combined with anterior cruciate ligament reconstruction. Am J Sports Med 2016;44(3): 593–601.
29. Rasmussen MT, Nitri M, Williams BT, et al. An in vitro robotic assessment of the anterolateral ligament, part 1: secondary role of the anterolateral ligament in the setting of an anterior cruciate ligament injury. Am J Sports Med 2016;44(3): 585–92.
30. Monaco E, Maestri B, Conteduca F, et al. Extra-articular ACL reconstruction and pivot shift: in vivo dynamic evaluation with navigation. Am J Sports Med 2014; 42(7):1669–74.

31. Slette EL, Mikula JD, Schon JM, et al. Biomechanical results of lateral extra-articular tenodesis procedures of the knee: a systematic review. Arthroscopy 2016;32(12):2592–611.
32. Schon JM, Moatshe G, Brady AW, et al. Anatomic anterolateral ligament reconstruction of the knee leads to overconstraint at any fixation angle. Am J Sports Med 2016;44(10):2546–56.
33. Dombrowski ME, Costello JM, Ohashi B, et al. Macroscopic anatomical, histological and magnetic resonance imaging correlation of the lateral capsule of the knee. Knee Surg Sports Traumatol Arthrosc 2016;24(9):2854–60.
34. Musahl V, Rahnemai-Azar AA, van Eck CF, et al. Anterolateral ligament of the knee, fact or fiction? Knee Surg Sports Traumatol Arthrosc 2016;24(1):2–3.
35. Rahnemai-Azar AA, Miller RM, Guenther D, et al. Structural properties of the anterolateral capsule and iliotibial band of the knee. Am J Sports Med 2016;44(4):892–7.
36. Guenther D, Rahnemai-Azar AA, Bell KM, et al. The anterolateral capsule of the knee behaves like a sheet of fibrous tissue. Am J Sports Med 2017;45(4):849–55.
37. Claes S, Vereecke E, Maes M, et al. Anatomy of the anterolateral ligament of the knee. J Anat 2013;223(4):321–8.
38. Smeets K, Slane J, Scheys L, et al. The anterolateral ligament has similar biomechanical and histologic properties to the inferior glenohumeral ligament. Arthroscopy 2017;1–8. http://dx.doi.org/10.1016/j.arthro.2017.01.038.
39. Capo J, Kaplan DJ, Fralinger DJ, et al. Ultrasonographic visualization and assessment of the anterolateral ligament. Knee Surg Sports Traumatol Arthrosc 2016;1–6. http://dx.doi.org/10.1007/s00167-016-4215-x.
40. Roessler PP, Schüttler KF, Heyse TJ, et al. The anterolateral ligament (ALL) and its role in rotational extra-articular stability of the knee joint: a review of anatomy and surgical concepts. Arch Orthop Trauma Surg 2016;136(3):305–13.
41. Levy I, Torzilli P, Gould J, et al. The effect of lateral meniscectomy on motion of the knee. J Bone Joint Surg Am 1989;71(3):401–6.
42. Levy I, Torzilli P, Warren RF. The effect of medial meniscectomy on anterior-posterior motion of the knee. J Bone Joint Surg Am 1982;64(6):883–8.
43. Musahl V, Citak M, O'Loughlin PF, et al. The effect of medial versus lateral meniscectomy on the stability of the anterior cruciate ligament-deficient knee. Am J Sports Med 2010;38(8):1591–7.
44. Shybut TB, Vega CE, Haddad J, et al. Effect of lateral meniscal root tear on the stability of the anterior cruciate ligament-deficient knee. Am J Sports Med 2015;43(4):905–11.
45. Hosseini A, Li J-S, Gill TJ, et al. Meniscus injuries alter the kinematics of knees with anterior cruciate ligament deficiency. Orthop J Sports Med 2014;2(8):1–8.
46. Musahl V, Rahnemai-Azar AA, Costello J, et al. The influence of meniscal and anterolateral capsular injury on knee laxity in patients with anterior cruciate ligament injuries. Am J Sports Med 2016;20(10):1–6.
47. Thompson W, Fu FH. The meniscus in the cruciate-deficient knee. Clin Sports Med 1993;12(4):771–96.
48. Wroble R, Grood E, Cummings J, et al. The role of the lateral extraarticular restraints in the anterior cruciate ligament-deficient knee. Am J Sports Med 1993;21(2):257–62.
49. Zantop T, Schumacher T, Diermann N, et al. Anterolateral rotational knee instability: Role of posterolateral structures. Arch Orthop Trauma Surg 2007;127(9):743–52.
50. Herbst E, Albers M, Burnham JM, et al. The anterolateral complex of the knee: a pictorial essay. Knee Surg Sports Traumatol Arthrosc 2017;25(4):1009–14.

Do We Need Extra-Articular Reconstructive Surgery?

Eivind Inderhaug, MD, MPH, PhD[a,b],
Andy Williams, FRCS(Orth), FFSEM[b,c,*]

KEYWORDS

- Anterolateral rotational instability • ALRI • ACL • Anterior cruciate ligament
- Lateral tenodeses • ALL • Anterolateral ligament

KEY POINTS

- Extra-articular anterolateral procedures have undergone a renaissance in combination with anterior cruciate ligament (ACL) reconstruction in selected cases.
- Biomechanical studies suggest that traditional lateral tenodeses are most efficient in restoring native knee kinematics in combined ACL and anterolateral injured knees.
- In optimizing technical details, such as graft path, tension, and angle of flexion at graft fixation, complications such as overconstraint can be avoided.
- There is a clear need for more high-level clinical evidence to support the routine use of lateral extra-articular procedures.

INTRODUCTION

Anterior cruciate ligament (ACL) tears are among the most common injuries in sports medicine, and although selected patients can function well with a nonoperative approach, surgical reconstruction is a mainstay in the treatment of these patients.[1,2] The surgical techniques have been evolving since the early twentieth century, using different approaches to eliminate the hallmark "giving way" symptoms of an ACL-deficient knee.[3]

Conflict of Interests: Editorial board member *Bone & Joint Journal*, trustee of Fortius Research and Education Foundation, director and shareholder in Fortius Clinic, director and shareholder in Innovate Orthopedics, Smith and Nephew part funding of a clinical fellow (A. Williams). Smith and Nephew research support, Smith and Nephew ad hoc payments for teaching (A. Williams, E. Inderhaug).
[a] Surgical Clinic, Haraldsplass Deaconess Hospital, Ulriksdal 8c, Bergen 5009, Norway; [b] Imperial College London, Exhibiton Road, London SW7 2AZ, UK; [c] Fortius Clinic, 17 Fitzhardige Street, London W1H 6EQ, UK
* Corresponding author. Fortius Clinic, 17 Fitzhardige Street, London W1H 6EQ, UK.
E-mail address: williams@fortiusclinic.com

Clin Sports Med 37 (2018) 61–73
http://dx.doi.org/10.1016/j.csm.2017.07.008
0278-5919/18/© 2017 Elsevier Inc. All rights reserved.

Former generations of knee surgeons used extra-articular tenodeses, originally often in isolation, for ACL insufficiency. A variety of eponymous techniques, like the Loose sling, Müller, Lemaire, Andrews, and MacIntosh procedures, were found effective in stabilizing the knee at the time of surgery and were widely used.[4–8] Clinical evaluations did, however, show variable outcomes and the tenodeses were suspected to cause lateral compartment osteoarthritis due to overconstraint.[9–11] With advance of reliable intra-articular ACL reconstruction, providing better clinical results and a less invasive approach, the use of extra-articular procedures declined and was continued in only a few centers and countries as an adjuvant procedure to modern intra-articular ACL reconstruction.[12–14]

Despite decades of research focusing on surgery for the ACL-deficient knee, there is still a significant failure rate after ACL reconstruction.[15,16] Findings of persistent rotational instability are not uncommon and suggest an inability of the intra-articular graft to normalize knee kinematics.[17–19] In response to this awareness, there has been a focus on optimizing the intra-articular graft function, such as in double-bundle ACL reconstruction, or changing graft tunnel positions. Recently, a renewed interest in anterolateral soft tissue structures, their clinical significance, and potential extra-articular procedures has provided a range of anatomic and biomechanical studies that give us new insights. The hope is to advance our understanding of anterolateral rotational instability (ALRI) and improve the results after surgery to avoid cases in which abnormal knee kinematics persist despite a technically well-done isolated intra-articular ACL reconstruction.

The aim of the current review was to make use of recent evidence, but keeping the historical perspective in mind, when discussing the rationale for applying extra-articular anterolateral procedures in combination with ACL reconstruction. Our intent is to display what is known on the topic, but also point out areas in which future investigation should provide us with new and currently unavailable knowledge.

WHY WERE EXTRA-ARTICULAR PROCEDURES LEFT BEHIND?

The extra-articular tenodeses were for many a mainstay in the treatment of ACL insufficiency from the late 1960s until the 1980s.[3,9] Most techniques did use some sort of graft from the iliotibial band (ITB), either free or left attached to the Gerdy tubercle. Although all these procedures aimed at, and to a large extent succeeded in, controlling ALRI, the dawning era of arthroscopically assisted ACL reconstruction saw a decline in their popularity. At this time, in 1989, an American Orthopedic Society for Sports Medicine consensus meeting was held to enlighten the future place of lateral extra-articular reconstructions (ER) in addressing ACL insufficiency.[11] A selected expert panel of well-renowned knee surgeons discussed a series of statements in light of available biomechanical and clinical evidence. Uniform conclusions were that *"extra-articular procedures (ER) were biomechanically inferior to intra-articular reconstruction (IR)"* and that *"ER was unable to restore normal biomechanics in an ACL-injured knee."* Regarding adjuvant use of ER with concomitant IR, little evidence was available. Interestingly, a common notion was that knee injuries leading to an ACL tear were understood to involve more than the intra-articular lesion (ie, anterolateral injuries) and that selected patients could benefit from a combined ER and IR approach. Although unanswered questions remained after the meeting, it did effectively end the era of extra-articular tenodeses in the United States. In European countries, such as the United Kingdom and France, a continued adjuvant use of the extra-articular procedures was thought to protect the intra-articular graft during healing, and has later provided us with important new knowledge on their effect.[14,20,21]

Although a range of studies (of variable scientific quality) at that time investigated the role of extra-articular procedures, some were more dominant than others. For example, O'Brien and colleagues,[22] reported on a series of 80 ACL reconstructions in which a patellar tendon reconstruction had been combined with a lateral sling at a minimum 2-year follow-up. No differences were found in clinical examination or in KT-1000 measurements. As a result, it was thought unnecessary to use additional ERs. Although this was one of the better studies of that time, the patients were not randomly allocated to treatments, and the retrospective manner of the study could have induced certain biases. Another influential study was a biomechanical investigation performed by Amis and Scammell.[23] In a controlled laboratory setting, knees were subject to an anterior drawer force that consistently resulted in an ACL tear. In that knee state, IR and ER were performed in isolation and in combination. Looking at Lachman, varus-valgus movements and rotational stability, the ER was clearly inferior to IR in restoring normal knee kinematics. Further, adding the ER to an IR made no difference to knee stability, leading to the conclusion that there was no biomechanical basis for ER whether in isolation or in combination with IR. In light of more recent studies, it does, however, seem that sole transection of the ACL will probably not fully replicate the ALRI that is seen in a "pivot shift": the hallmark clinical sign of ACL-deficient patients. Several studies have suggested that an anterolateral lesion is a prerequisite for the pivot shift to occur.[24–26]

In summary, there were some clear limitations in studies, and the culture at the time that catalyzed the shift to the modern "intra-articular paradigm" in approaching ACL surgery, and a reevaluation of the place for extra-articular tenodeses, therefore, seems warranted.

IS THERE SUCH A THING AS AN ANTEROLATERAL INJURY IN ANTERIOR CRUCIATE LIGAMENT TEARS?

There are several mechanisms of injury that may lead to an ACL tear, and concomitant injuries, such as meniscal tears or injuries to collateral ligaments.[27,28]Activities that include sudden decelerations and cutting maneuvers are more risk prone, but injury mechanisms vary from sport to sport.[29] Levine and colleagues[30] induced ACL injury in 15 of 17 knees by the combination of tibial internal rotation, valgus force, anterior tibial translation, and axial compression. This has been proposed as the most common combination of forces that will cause the ACL to tear and it certainly fits well with the classic lateral compartment pattern of bone bruising on the mid-femur and posterior tibia. Knowing that anterolateral structures have recently been shown to play a role in controlling internal rotation in the knee, it is likely that a forceful internal torque is involved when these are injured.[26,31,32]

Some of the most reliable knowledge of incidence and distribution of anterolateral injuries are from studies that have performed open exploration during surgery. Terry and colleagues,[33] in a series of 82 patients undergoing ACL reconstruction within 3 weeks of injury, found lesions of anterolateral soft tissue structures in 93% of cases. The most common sites of injury were deep layers of ITB (82%), proximal/distal capsulo-osseous layers of ITB (71%), mid capsulo-osseous layer of ITB (29%), and the superficial layer of the ITB (9%). In a more recent study, Ferretti and colleagues[34] explored a series of 60 patients who underwent acute ACL surgery (less than a week from injury). Fifty-four of 60 patients were found to have some sort of macroscopic soft tissue tear. Grading of the anterolateral lesions/injuries was in that study focused on the recently described "anterolateral" ligament (ALL), and these findings were therefore not directly comparable to that from the former study.

Furthermore, a range of studies performing radiologic assessment of anterolateral injuries has been published. Traditionally, the eponymous Segond fracture has been thought of as a hallmark sign of ACL, and anterolateral injuries, representing an avulsion of the ITB.[35] But when looking at the relatively small-sized patient series published that have showcased this injury (from 9–29 patients), it is clear that the sensitivity of this sign in detecting combined injuries must be poor.[35–38] More recent ultrasound and MRI studies have displayed a somewhat higher incidence of concomitant injuries to anterolateral soft tissues in those diagnosed with an ACL tear. Mansour and colleagues,[39] found signs of ITB injuries in 56% of patients on MRI scans, whereas Hartigan and colleagues[40] described an incidence of ALL injuries from 26% to 62%. In the latter study, an intrarater agreement of only 0.54 was seen between 2 trained radiologists, leading the investigators to conclude that current radiological assessment of anterolateral structure integrity is at best unreliable. At present, differences in the understanding and classification of anterolateral structures are major barriers for uniform and accurate radiological diagnosis, making comparison across studies difficult. Further work toward a common consensus in the anatomic description is paramount if we are to advance in the field of diagnostics and reach a common understanding of these injuries.

Although a high incidence of concomitant anterolateral injuries is found in an early phase after the initial knee trauma leading to an ACL tear, very little is known about how these injuries, and any related laxities, will evolve over time. On one hand, one could speculate whether there is a healing potential, such as seen in medial collateral ligament injuries, that will eliminate any excessive laxity over time.[41] On the other hand, when considering studies showing residual instability after ACL reconstruction, one might speculate that these laxities persist over time.

IS THERE ANY EVIDENCE FOR AN ADDITIONAL EFFECT OF ANTEROLATERAL PROCEDURES?

Looking back at a range of clinical studies that have reported on outcomes after ACL reconstruction combined with anterolateral procedures, a heterogeneous picture is seen. With differences in the surgical techniques (both ACL reconstruction and tenodeses), retrospective designs, and a large variability in methods for outcome evaluation, it is hard to assimilate these results. Studies like those from Roth and colleagues,[42] O'Brien and colleagues,[43] and Strum and colleagues[44] have found no additional effect of a combined approach, and therefore conclude that intra-articular ACL reconstruction is sufficient on its own when addressing the ACL-deficient knee. Other reports, like those from Vadalà and colleagues,[45] Zaffagnini and colleagues,[46] and Bignozzi and colleagues,[47] have found beneficial effects of the added procedure, including less anterior translation at time zero, improved International Knee Documentation Committee (IKDC) subjective score and a reduction in pivot shift at the time of follow-up, all in favor of the combined approach. A recent meta-analysis by Hewison and colleagues[10] aimed to determine whether the addition of a lateral extra-articular tenodesis (LET) would provide greater control of rotational laxity and improved clinical outcomes as compared with ACL reconstruction alone. Although the meta-analysis did not find any superiority in subjective outcomes, an overall reduction in pivot shift in favor of a combined approach was seen. Most of the 29 studies included in the review were found to have low sample size and a poor methodological quality.

Some of the recent work providing new insights has been biomechanical studies using cadaveric knees. Kittl and colleagues[48] investigated length change patterns in a variety of anatomic structures and potential anterolateral procedures. Presuming that relatively isometric graft behavior, meaning a minimal graft length change throughout the knee range of motion, is desirable, some interesting findings were seen. Although the tested structures/procedures had a wide variety of elongation patterns, 2 factors did reliably predict an isometric graft behavior: a graft path deep to the lateral collateral ligament (LCL) and femoral graft insertion proximal/posterior to the lateral epicondyle. A key for these findings is thought to be a "pulley effect" of the LCL that facilitates this beneficial behavior. It may be that this better reproduces the curved attachment of the deep capsule–osseous ITB to the lateral knee. Kittl and colleagues[26] also studied the relative importance of lateral soft tissue structures in resisting anterior tibial translation, internal rotation, and combined internal rotation and anterior tibial translation. This study found the ITB to be the most important restraining structure (**Fig. 1**). The ACL itself was important only in full knee extension. The ALL was, however, not found to be of particular importance.

Of the relatively few studies that have compared the performance of a selection of anterolateral procedures, only 2 have done so in knees with a combined ACL and anterolateral injury; prior cadaver studies simply divided the ACL to mimic the ACL-deficient state and did not create an anterolateral lesion. Spencer and colleagues[49] performed an ALL reconstruction using braided suture tape and a modified Lemaire procedure using a 1-cm strip of the ITB. The ALL procedure used in that study was unable to restore normal internal rotation resistance, whereas the Lemaire procedure had favorable effects showing significant improvements in rotational control. Similarly, Inderhaug and colleagues[50] reported on a selection of procedures in their biomechanical work. In that study, an anatomic ACL reconstruction was found to leave residual laxity if used as the only procedure in a combined injured knee. Next,

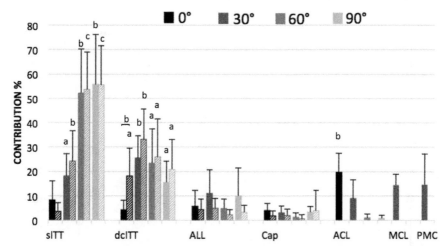

Fig. 1. Displaying the relative contribution of tested structures in restraining a 5-Nm internal rotation torque at 0, 30, 60, and 90° of knee flexion. Cross-hatched areas indicate results from the ACL-deficient groups, and solid bars indicate those with the ACL intact. Results shown are mean ± SD (n = 8). Statistically significant changes from the initial knee state (brackets indicate significant difference between ACL intact vs deficient): [a]$P<.05$, [b]$P<.01$, and [c]$P<.001$. Cap, antero-lateral capsule; dcITT, deep and capsulo-osseous layer of the iliotibial tract; MCL, medial collateral ligament; PMC, posteromedial corner; sITT, superficial layer of the iliotibial tract. (*From* Kittl C, El-Daou H, Athwal KK, et al. The role of the anterolateral structures and the ACL in controlling laxity of the intact and ACL-deficient knee. Am J Sports Med 2016;44:351, with permission; and *Courtesy of* Sage Publications, Thousand Oaks, CA, with permission.)

an ALL reconstruction, a Lemaire tenodesis, and a MacIntosh tenodesis were performed in a randomized order. The latter 2 procedures did restore a normal kinematic pattern, whereas the ALL procedure had no effect on knee stability (**Fig. 2**). Another important finding was that applying 20 N of graft tension (2 kg) was enough to restore normal knee kinematics. If a higher 40 N (4 kg) was applied, a tendency, although not statistically significant, to overconstraint (ie, a loss of internal rotation) was seen.

Besides the role of anterolateral procedures in abolishing any excessive knee laxity, there seems to be another potential benefit from applying a combined approach at ACL reconstruction. Engebretsen and colleagues[51] studied not only knee joint motion but also graft forces in combined intra-articular and extra-articular procedures. Their results displayed that adding an extra-articular graft would lead to an off-loading of the intra-articular graft by approximately 43%. The same findings were confirmed by Draganich and colleagues,[5] as load sharing was seen between the intra-articular and extra-articular grafts during rotational and translation stresses. Based on these findings, one could hypothesize a beneficial protective effect on the intra-articular graft during early rehabilitation, particularly important for patients returning early to strenuous activity, such as professional athletes.

COMPLICATIONS OF ANTEROLATERAL PROCEDURES?

A common fear with the extra-articular procedures is the perceived risk of osteoarthritis due to overconstraint of the lateral compartment (see previously in this article). Although this notion is much discussed, and frequently cited, there is very little evidence to establish such a link.[9,11] It is also important to note that a dramatic change in postoperative rehabilitation has taken place over the past few decades.[52,53] Most

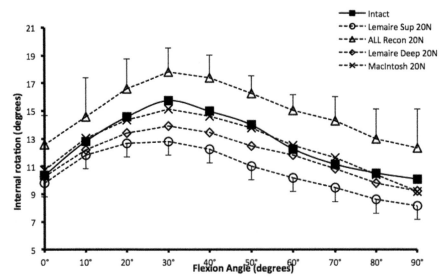

Fig. 2. Internal rotation under 5-Nm internal torque for intact, Lemaire superficial (Lemaire Sup), Lemaire deep, MacIntosh, and ALL reconstructions (ALL Recon), all with 20-N tensioning (n = 8). Values represent mean ± SD. (*From* Inderhaug E, Stephen JM, Williams A, et al. Biomechanical comparison of anterolateral procedures combined with anterior cruciate ligament reconstruction. Am J Sports Med 2017;45(2):350, with permission; and *Courtesy of* Sage Publishing, Thousand Oaks, CA, with permission.)

importantly, a shift from postoperative immobilization (sometimes using a cast) to early mobilization has probably reduced the risk of fixed contractures of knee rotation that could overload lateral compartment cartilage.

Samuelson and colleagues[54] investigated the effect of a tenodesis performed with 2 different graft tensions in a series of cadaveric knees. The tension was varied between 0 N and 22 N at graft fixation. A tendency of overconstraining the knee, most pronounced with the higher graft tension, was found both in anterior translation and internal rotation. The investigators therefore suggested that the surgeon could affect the kinematic pattern of the knee by adjusting the tensioning of the tenodesis. In another study, Inderhaug and colleagues,[55] applied intra-articular pressure sensors to map any changes in cartilage pressures resulting from such overconstraint. Graft tensions of 20 N and 80 N were used in a MacIntosh tenodesis and pressure changes as well as kinematic responses were recorded in knees that were loaded to mimic weight bearing. Only the latter, much higher, 80-N tension resulted in significant increases in contact pressure because the knee was pulled into external rotation. This overconstraint could, however, be avoided if the knee was held in neutral rotation (as opposed to being left free hanging) at the time of graft tensioning and fixation. Yet another study by Schon and colleagues[56] found overconstraint when applying an ALL reconstruction with an anatomic ACL reconstruction. In that study, an 88-N graft tension was applied when fixing the graft. The current authors would question the effectiveness of the ALL reconstruction when as much as 88 N (8.8 kg of pull) is needed to achieve a kinematic effect. It is perhaps not surprising when the ALL is a relatively small and variably described ligament that contributes only little to resisting anterior tibial translation and internal rotation, a reconstruction of such a structure could have an effect only if tensioned highly. It does seem more appropriate to use one of the formerly discussed tenodeses techniques that could reliably restore normal knee kinematics using only 20 N of graft tensioning (MacIntosh or Lemaire), and thereby avoid any risk of overconstraint.[50] Finally, all of the previously mentioned studies reported on results at time zero after surgery and do, therefore, not account for changes in tension that might happen due to stretching of the graft in the early postoperative rehabilitation. This could perhaps further reduce the chance of overconstraint after a lateral extra-articular procedure. Nevertheless, with the renewed use of these procedures, it is important that proper and prolonged clinical follow-up evaluations of these studies are undertaken.

Other adverse events have been suggested to included donor site morbidity and risk of postoperative infection. In the classic study by O'Brien and colleagues,[43] 40% of patients were reported to have pain or swelling over the site of the "lateral sling" at their follow-up 2 years after surgery. According to a recent review, no other studies found the same tendency,[10] but this may simply mean that the studies concerned simply did not report this issue. For ITB-based LET, some local thickening is logical, as one layer of ITB will become 2 or 3 at the end of the procedure (**Fig. 3**).

The risk of septic arthritis was investigated by Sonnery-Cottet and colleagues[57] in a group of 1957 patients who had undergone ACL reconstruction. Two variables were found to relate to a higher incidence of septic arthritis: (1) being a professional athlete and (2) having a combined lateral tenodesis. A significant correlation between these 2 factors suggested a possible confounding effect. The investigators therefore concluded that the primary risk factor was being a professional athlete rather than having the conjunct lateral tenodesis. The current authors have not seen such a trend in their own practice, but do occasionally notice a postoperative hematoma after performing a lateral tenodesis. If being meticulous when harvesting the proximal part of the central ITB graft, one can, however, avoid lesions to the superior genicular artery

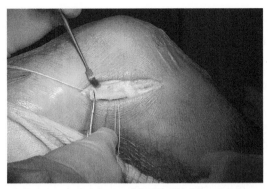

Fig. 3. A Lemaire tenodesis using a midstrip of the iliotibial band that is tunneled deep to the lateral collateral ligament and fixated just distal and posterior to the lateral epicondyle. Graft fixation is, in this case, performed using a suture anchor. The remaining graft is then sutured back onto itself before closure of the iliotibial band. (*Courtesy of* Eivind Inderhaug, MD, MPH, PhD, Surgical Clinic, Haraldsplass Deaconess Hospital, Bergen, Norway.)

that is in close proximity to the harvesting site and is the likely reason for this hematoma.

CURRENT TREATMENT RECOMMENDATIONS

Although the past 2 decades have seen many studies and much effort spent on developing and fine-tuning the intra-articular ACL reconstruction, the role of extra-articular lateral procedures are now being heavily debated.[58–60] Along with the realization that formerly unaddressed meniscal injuries, such as root lesions and the ramp lesion, could have contributed to residual laxity after an ACL reconstruction, there seems to be an evolving rationale for anterolateral procedures in addressing excessive ALRI.[61,62] There is, however, little hard evidence that gives clear indications for their use. A recent article, consulting global experts on the field, saw a unison agreement that these procedures do have a place in current ACL surgery.[63] Most of those questioned reported using some modification of the Lemaire tenodesis (see **Fig. 3**). Other procedures included versions of ALL reconstructions and a combined intra-articular and extra-articular hamstring procedure. The use of a combined approach in primary ACL reconstructions was reported to range from 5% to 80%, whereas they were used in up to 100% of revision surgery cases. The reality is that there is no "evidence-based" approach, and most surgeons regularly undertaking ERs use them in any case that is felt to be at higher risk of intra-articular graft re-rupture.

At present, there seems to be 2 main reasons for applying a combined approach when performing surgery in an ACL-injured knee. First, given that anterolateral structures have been found to restrain internal rotation of the knee, an important component of ALRI, and underpinned by the finding that these structures seem to be frequently injured when the ACL is torn, patients with a high-grade pivot shift, for example, IKDC grade II or III, should be considered for a combined approach. Second, given that an anterolateral procedure might offer load sharing between intra-articular and extra-articular grafts, there might be a role for a combined approach in patients who are returning to sports at a high level, such as professional athletes. These are known to have a higher risk of reinjury and will expose their knee to greater forces earlier in the postoperative rehabilitation.[64,65] Additionally, there seems to be a common agreement about a lower threshold for applying the combined approach in patients undergoing revision surgery. Other proposed indications include juvenile patients (in whom ER grafts can be fixed distal to the growth plate by using intraoperative fluoroscopy), and those with ligament hyperlaxity and hyperextension excess.

FUTURE RESEARCH

With the common aim of improving patient outcomes and reducing the number of failed ACL reconstructions, there is a clear need for further work in several areas related to the use of anterolateral procedures. First, more fine-tuned diagnostic tools must be sought if aiming to differentiate between intra-articular and extra-articular lesions of the knee, not only with regard to radiological modalities, but also to aid more accurate clinical examination, to help define when ER is needed. Furthermore, technical details on how to best perform an extra-articular procedure are crucial if aiming to reduce adverse effects and optimize the surgery. An example is a recent biomechanical work that investigated which angle of flexion should be applied at graft tensioning.[66] That study found that a modified Lemaire procedure did normalize knee kinematics independent of this variable, but with an ALL procedure, the most favorable kinematic pattern was found if the graft was tensioned at full extension. Furthermore, additional high-quality randomized controlled studies are needed to investigate the clinical outcome after isolated ACL reconstruction versus a combined approach.

SUMMARY

The present review discussed the role anterolateral procedures have in conjunction with modern ACL reconstruction in light of current available evidence. There seems to be a renaissance of modifications of formerly well-described ITB-based tenodeses, such as the Lemaire procedure, and a rise in the popularity of the more recently described ALL reconstructions. Biomechanical studies have found the LET to have favorable effects that help normalize kinematics in combined ACL and anterolateral injuries, whereas ALL reconstructions do not seem be as effective. Only if a very high 88-N graft tension was applied did the ALL deal with excess laxity, but at the price of a clearly overconstrained knee. Technical details, such as graft tension, flexion angle at graft fixation, and knee position at graft fixation all act synergistically toward achieving the optimal effect of these procedures. Controlling rotation of the knee at graft fixation to prevent fixed external rotation seems especially important to avoid increases in lateral compartment chondral pressures. The use of a combined approach is cautiously recommended in a selected group of patients (eg, high-degree rotational instability and high-demand patient) but there is a clear need for better diagnostic tools to decide when to use them and high-level clinical studies that investigate the additional effect over isolated ACL reconstruction in the longer term.

REFERENCES

1. Delincé P, Ghafil D. Anterior cruciate ligament tears: conservative or surgical treatment? A critical review of the literature. Knee Surg Sports Traumatol Arthrosc 2011;20:48–61.
2. Smith TO, Postle K, Penny F, et al. Is reconstruction the best management strategy for anterior cruciate ligament rupture? A systematic review and meta-analysis comparing anterior cruciate ligament reconstruction versus non-operative treatment. Knee 2014;21:462–70.

3. Burnett QM, Fowler PJ. Reconstruction of the anterior cruciate ligament: historical overview. Orthop Clin North Am 1985;16:143–57.

4. Losee RE, Johnson TR, Southwick WO. Anterior subluxation of the lateral tibial plateau. A diagnostic test and operative repair. J Bone Joint Surg Am 1978;60: 1015–30.

5. Draganich LF, Reider B, Miller PR. An in vitro study of the Müller anterolateral femorotibial ligament tenodesis in the anterior cruciate ligament deficient knee. Am J Sports Med 1989;17:357–62.

6. Lemaire M. Ruptures anciennes du ligament croisé antérieur du genou. J Chir 1967;93:311–20.

7. Andrews JR, Sanders R. A "mini-reconstruction" technique in treating anterolateral rotatory instability (ALRI). Clin Orthop Relat Res 1983;172:93–6.

8. Ireland J, Trickey EL. Macintosh tenodesis for anterolateral instability of the knee. J Bone Joint Surg Br 1980;62:340–5.

9. Dodds AL, Gupte CM, Neyret P, et al. Extra-articular techniques in anterior cruciate ligament reconstruction: a literature review. J Bone Joint Surg Br 2011;93: 1440–8.

10. Hewison CE, Tran MN, Kaniki N, et al. Lateral extra-articular tenodesis reduces rotational laxity when combined with anterior cruciate ligament reconstruction: a systematic review of the literature. Arthroscopy 2015;31:2022–34.

11. Ferretti A. Extra-articular reconstruction in the anterior cruciate ligament deficient knee: a commentary. Joints 2014;2:41–7.

12. Marcacci M, Zaffagnini S, Giordano G, et al. Anterior cruciate ligament reconstruction associated with extra-articular tenodesis: a prospective clinical and radiographic evaluation with 10- to 13-year follow-up. Am J Sports Med 2009; 37:707–14.

13. Neyret P, Palomo JR, Donell ST, et al. Extra-articular tenodesis for anterior cruciate ligament rupture in amateur skiers. Br J Sports Med 1994;28:31–4.

14. Acquitter Y, Hulet C, Locker J, et al. Intérêt d'une plastie extra-articulaire dans le traitement des laxités antérieures chroniques du gnou par une autogreffe de tendon rotulien. Rev Chir Orthop 2003;89:413–22.

15. Crawford SN, Waterman BR, Lubowitz JH. Long-term failure of anterior cruciate ligament reconstruction. Arthroscopy 2013;29:1566–71.

16. Inderhaug E, Raknes S, Østvold T, et al. Increased revision rate with posterior tibial tunnel placement after using the 70-degree tibial guide in ACL reconstruction. Knee Surg Sports Traumatol Arthrosc 2017;25(1):152–8.

17. Logan MC. Tibiofemoral kinematics following successful anterior cruciate ligament reconstruction using dynamic multiple resonance imaging. Am J Sports Med 2004;32:984–92.

18. Tashman S, Kolowich P, Collon D, et al. Dynamic function of the ACL-reconstructed knee during running. Clin Orthop Relat Res 2007;454:66–73.

19. Georgoulis AD, Ristanis S, Moriati CO, et al. ACL injury and reconstruction: clincial related in vivo biomechanics. Orthop Traumatol Surg Res 2010;96:119–28.

20. Lerat JL, Mandrino A, Besse JL, et al. Influence d'une ligmentoplastie extra-articulaire externe sur les résultats de la reconstruction du ligament croisé antérieur avec le tendon rotulien, avec quatreans de recul. Rev Chir Orthop 1997;83: 591–601.

21. Rackemann S, Robinson A, Dandy DJ. Reconstruction of the anterior cruciate ligament with an intra-articular patellar tendon graft and an extra-articular tenodesis. Results after six years. J Bone Joint Surg Br 1991;73:368–73.

22. O'Brien SJ, Warren RF, Pavlov H, et al. Reconstruction of the chronically insuffi-cient anterior cruciate ligament with the central third of the patellar ligament. J Bone Joint Surg Am 1991;73:278–86.
23. Amis AA, Scammell BE. Biomechanics of intra-articular and extra-articular recon-struction of the anterior cruciate ligament. J Bone Joint Surg Br 1993;75:812–7.
24. Hughston JC, Andrews JR, Cross MJ, et al. Classification of knee ligament insta-bilities. Part II. The lateral compartment. J Bone Joint Surg Am 1976;58:173–9.
25. Tanaka M, Vyas D, Moloney G, et al. What does it take to have a high-grade pivot shift? Knee Surg Sports Traumatol Arthrosc 2012;20:737–42.
26. Kittl C, El-Daou H, Athwal KK, et al. The role of the anterolateral structures and the ACL in controlling laxity of the intact and ACL-deficient knee. Am J Sports Med 2016;44:345–54.
27. Ahlden M, Samuelsson K, Sernert N, et al. The Swedish National Anterior Cruciate Ligament Register. Am J Sports Med 2012;40:2230–5.
28. Rotterud JH, Sivertsen EA, Forssblad M, et al. Effect of meniscal and focal carti-lage lesions on patient-reported outcome after anterior cruciate ligament recon-struction: a Nationwide Cohort Study From Norway and Sweden of 8476 patients with 2-year follow-up. Am J Sports Med 2013;41:535–43.
29. Hughes G, Watkins J. A risk-factor model for anterior cruciate ligament injury. Sports Med 2006;36(5):411–28.
30. Levine JW, Kiapour AM, Quatman CE, et al. Clinically relevant injury patterns after an anterior cruciate ligament injury provide insight into injury mechanisms. Am J Sports Med 2013;41:385–95.
31. Wroble RR, Grood ES, Cummings JS, et al. The role of the lateral extraarticular restraints in the anterior cruciate ligament-deficient knee. Am J Sports Med 1993;21:257–63.
32. Rasmussen MT, Nitri M, Williams BT, et al. An in vitro robotic assessment of the anterolateral ligament, part 1: secondary role of the anterolateral ligament in the setting of an anterior cruciate ligament injury. Am J Sports Med 2016;44:585–92.
33. Terry GC, Norwood LA, Hughston JC, et al. How iliotibial tract injuries of the knee combine with acute anterior cruciate ligament tears to influence abnormal ante-rior tibial displacement. Am J Sports Med 1993;21:55–60.
34. Ferretti A, Monaco E, Fabbri M, et al. Prevalence and classification of injuries of anterolateral complex in acute anterior cruciate ligament tears. Arthroscopy 2017;33:147–51.
35. Goldman AB, Pavlov H, Rubenstein D. The Segond fracture of the proximal tibia: a small avulsion that reflects major ligamentous damage. AJR Am J Roentgenol 1988;151:1163–7.
36. Claes S, Luyckx T, Vereecke E, et al. The Segond fracture: a bony injury of the anterolateral ligament of the knee. Arthroscopy 2014;30:1475–82.
37. Hess T, Rupp S, Hopf T, et al. Lateral tibial avulsion fractures and disruptions to the anterior cruciate ligament. A clinical study of their incidence and correlation. Clin Orthop Relat Res 1994;303:193–7.
38. Campos JC, Chung CB, Lektrakul N. Pathogenesis of the Segond fracture: anatomic and MR imaging evidence of an iliotibial tract or anterior oblique band avulsion. Radiology 2001;219:381–6.
39. Mansour R, Yoong P, McKean D, et al. The iliotibial band in acute knee trauma: patterns of injury on MR imaging. Skeletal Radiol 2014;43:1369–75.
40. Hartigan DE, Carrol KW, Kosarek FJ, et al. Visibility of anterolateral ligament tears in anterior cruciate ligament. Arthroscopy 2016;32:2061–5.

41. Woo SL, Vogrin TM, Abramowitch SD. Healing and repair of ligament injuries in the knee. J Am Acad Orthop Surg 2000;8:364–72.

42. Roth JH, Kennedy JC, Lockstadt H, et al. Intra-articular reconstruction of the anterior cruciate ligament with and without extra-articular supplementation by transfer of the biceps femoris tendon. J Bone Joint Surg Am 1987;69:275–8.

43. O'Brien SJ, Warren RF, Wickiewicz TL, et al. The iliotibial band lateral sling procedure and its effect on the results of anterior cruciate ligament reconstruction. Am J Sports Med 1991;19:21–4.

44. Strum GM, Fox JM, Ferkel RD, et al. Intraarticular versus intraarticular and extra-articular reconstruction for chronic anterior cruciate ligament instability. Clin Orthop Relat Res 1989;245:188–98.

45. Vadalà AP, Iorio R, De Carli A, et al. An extra-articular procedure improves the clinical outcome in anterior cruciate ligament reconstruction with hamstrings in female athletes. Int Orthop 2012;37:187–92.

46. Zaffagnini S, Bruni D, Russo A, et al. ST/G ACL reconstruction: double strand plus extra-articular sling vs double bundle, randomized study at 3-year follow-up. Scand J Med Sci Sports 2008;18:573–81.

47. Bignozzi S, Zaffagnini S, Lopomo N, et al. Does a lateral plasty control coupled translation during antero-posterior stress in single-bundle ACL reconstruction? An in vivo study. Knee Surg Sports Traumatol Arthrosc 2008;17:65–70.

48. Kittl C, Halewood C, Stephen JM, et al. Length change patterns in the lateral extra-articular structures of the knee and related reconstructions. Am J Sports Med 2014;43:354–62.

49. Spencer L, Burkhart TA, Tran MN, et al. Biomechanical analysis of simulated clinical testing and reconstruction of the anterolateral ligament of the knee. Am J Sports Med 2015;43:2189–97.

50. Inderhaug E, Stephen JM, Williams A, et al. Biomechanical comparison of anterolateral procedures combined with anterior cruciate ligament reconstruction. Am J Sports Med 2017;45(2):347–54.

51. Engebretsen L, Lew WD, Lewis JL, et al. The effect of an iliotibial tenodesis on intra-articular graft forces and knee joint motion. Am J Sports Med 1990;18:169–76.

52. Donald Shelbourne K, Klotz C. What I have learned about the ACL: utilizing a progressive rehabilitation scheme to achieve total knee symmetry after anterior cruciate ligament reconstruction. J Orthop Sci 2006;11:318–25.

53. Howell SM, Hull ML. Aggressive rehabilitation using hamstring tendons: graft construct, tibial tunnel placement, fixation properties, and clinical outcome. Am J Knee Surg 1998;11(2):120–7.

54. Samuelson M, Draganich LF, Zhou X, et al. The effects of knee reconstruction on combined anterior cruciate ligament and anterolateral capsular deficiencies. Am J Sports Med 1996;24:492–7.

55. Inderhaug E, Stephen JM, El-Daou H, et al. The effects of anterolateral tenodesis on tibiofemoral contact pressures and kinematics. Am J Sports Med 2017. http://dx.doi.org/10.1177/0363546517717260.

56. Schon JM, Moatshe G, Brady AW, et al. Anatomic anterolateral ligament reconstruction of the knee leads to overconstraint at any fixation angle. Am J Sports Med 2016;44(10):2546–56.

57. Sonnery-Cottet B, Archbold P, Zayni R, et al. Prevalence of septic arthritis after anterior cruciate ligament reconstruction among professional athletes. Am J Sports Med 2011;39:2371–6.

58. Lubowitz JH. Editorial commentary: knee lateral extra-articular tenodesis. Arthroscopy 2015;31:2035.

59. Rossi MJ. Editorial commentary: addressing the anterolateral side of an anterior cruciate ligament-deficient knee: the controversy is getting even more interesting. Arthroscopy 2016;32:2048–9.
60. Noyes FR. Editorial commentary: lateral extra-articular reconstructions with anterior cruciate ligament surgery: are these operative procedures supported by in vitro biomechanical studies? Arthroscopy 2016;32:2612–5.
61. LaPrade RF, Matheny LM, Moulton SG, et al. Posterior meniscal root repairs: outcomes of an anatomic transtibial pull-out technique. Am J Sports Med 2017;45: 884–91.
62. Stephen JM, Halewood C, Kittl C, et al. Posteromedial meniscocapsular lesions increase tibiofemoral joint laxity with anterior cruciate ligament deficiency, and their repair reduces laxity. Am J Sports Med 2016;44:400–8.
63. Musahl V. Contributions of the anterolateral complex and the anterolateral ligament to rotatory knee stability in the setting of ACL injury: a roundtable discussion. Knee Surg Sports Traumatol Arthrosc 2017;25(4):997–1008.
64. Grindem H, Snyder-Mackler L, Moksnes H, et al. Simple decision rules can reduce reinjury risk by 84% after ACL reconstruction: the Delaware-Oslo ACL cohort study. Br J Sports Med 2016;50:804–8.
65. Wiggins AJ, Grandhi RK, Schneider DK, et al. Risk of secondary injury in younger athletes after anterior cruciate ligament reconstruction: a systematic review and meta-analysis. Am J Sports Med 2016;44:1861–76.
66. Inderhaug E, Stephen JM, Williams A, et al. Anterolateral tenodesis or ALL reconstruction: effect of flexion angle at graft fixation when combined with ACL reconstruction. Am J Sports Med 2017. in press.

Anterolateral Ligament Reconstruction or Extra-Articular Tenodesis: Why and When?

CrossMark

Manoj Mathew, MS(ortho), FRACS, Aad Dhollander, MD, PT, PhD,
Alan Getgood, MPhil, MD, FRCS (Tr&Orth), DipSEM*

KEYWORDS

- Anterior cruciate ligament (ACL) • ACL reconstruction
- Lateral extra-articular tenodesis (LET) • Anterolateral ligament (ALL)
- ALL reconstruction

KEY POINTS

- Residual rotational laxity after anterior cruciate ligament (ACL) reconstruction is a key determinant of outcomes, including patient satisfaction and return to sport.
- There is a renewed interest in combining extra-articular reconstruction techniques with intra-articular ACL reconstruction, as surgeons aim to provide consistent restoration of function including rotational control in a diverse cohort of patients.
- The currently used extra-articular augmentation techniques include lateral extra-articular tenodesis or anterolateral ligament reconstructions.
- Clinical superiority of one augmentation technique over the other is not yet proven and our technique is based on evidence from currently available biomechanical studies.

INTRODUCTION

The aim of an optimally performed anterior cruciate ligament (ACL) reconstruction is to restore both the anteroposterior and rotational stability observed in an ACL intact knee. Patient satisfaction, overall knee function, return to sports, and functional scores correlate more with restoration of rotational stability than translational stability,[1,2] making it a key short-term to mid-term goal. Long-term concerns pertaining to the risk of posttraumatic osteoarthritis have also been raised in the rotationally unstable knee.[3]

With the evolution of surgical techniques, including single and double-bundle options, improvements in rotational stability has been observed.[4–7] However, despite technical improvements, high rates of positive pivot shift tests continue to be observed in both contemporary techniques of single as well as double-bundle surgery,

Disclosure: The authors have no conflict of interest in regards to the content of this work.
The Fowler Kennedy Sport Medicine Clinic, University of Western Ontario, London, Ontario, Canada
* Corresponding author.
E-mail address: alan.getgood@uwo.ca

as tabled in a recent meta-analysis by Desai and colleagues.[8] A navigation study by Ferretti and colleagues[9] found that the addition of the posterolateral bundle to the anteromedial bundle in a double-bundle reconstruction did not significantly improve the rotational control, and that a well-positioned single bundle had similar rotational control. Furthermore, a computer-navigated cadaveric sectioning study by Monaco and colleagues[10] found that the posterolateral bundle did not significantly control rotation, but that sectioning of the anterolateral capsule resulted in a significant change in rotation.

These and several other studies have led to a resurgence of interest in methods new and old that could be used to augment the extra-articular structures of the anterolateral corner of the knee, and thus provide added rotational stability in ACL reconstructions.

THE ANTEROLATERAL SOFT TISSUE RESTRAINTS

The anterolateral soft tissue restraints to abnormal internal rotation in an ACL-deficient knee include the anterolateral capsule incorporating the anterolateral ligament (ALL), the iliotibial band (ITB), including the deep Kaplan fiber attachment to the distal femur, the menisci, and its capsular attachments.

In 1879, the French surgeon Paul Segond[11] described a "pearly, resistant, fibrous band inserting on the anterolateral aspect of the proximal tibia," while describing the eponymous fracture that is now considered pathognomonic of an ACL injury. Hughston and colleagues[12] identified that the "middle third of the lateral capsular ligament" was technically strong, attached proximally to the lateral epicondyle and distally to the tibial joint margin. Of cases with "anterolateral rotational instability," they identified it to be torn in 5 acute clinical cases (4 of whom had an ACL injury) and lax in 20 chronic cases (15 with an ACL injury). Recent MRI studies have also documented ALL injuries in 46% to 79% of ACL injuries.[13,14] As shown in recent studies, including one performed at our center, the ALL is a capsular thickening present within the substance of the anterolateral capsule with collagen bundle arrangements similar to that in a ligamentous structure.[15,16] The femoral attachment of the ALL has been described to be somewhat variable in position, inserting either posterior-proximal or anterior-distal to the femoral origin of the fibular collateral ligament (FCL) and the tibial attachment is located halfway between the Gerdy tubercle and the FCL insertion into the fibular head.[15–18] The ALL tibial attachment seen in cadaver specimens has been shown to match the radiologic location of clinically observed Segond fractures.[13,17] Following observations that the ALL with an origin posterior and proximal to the FCL is relatively isometric (although its length increases with flexion), compared with a distal and anterior origin,[19,20] the currently adopted femoral attachment site in ALL reconstructive procedures is the proximal posterior location. Experimental studies indicate that the ALL contributes to stability against internal rotation, particularly in flexion angles beyond 30°, reaching a peak contribution between 60 and 75° of flexion, with significant effect continuing beyond that.[10,21,22] This change of stability with flexion could be secondary to several reasons, including the effect of the ALL increasingly becoming taut with flexion as well as its orientation changing from being nearly perpendicular to the joint at full extension to being more parallel as flexion angle increases, resulting in a better vector for rotational control.

The deep part of the ITB and its complex distal femoral attachment also significantly contribute to anterolateral stability. Kaplan[23] observed that deep attachment of the ITB through the lateral intermuscular septum to the lateral femoral condyle resulted in it functioning like a ligament through its femoral and tibial bone insertions. Terry and colleagues[24] described the "capsulo-osseous layer" of the deep part of the ITB, which they initially named the anterolateral ligament (which should not be mistaken for the currently described ALL). This is anatomically a separate layer located superficial to the ALL and anterolateral capsule, and has its origin at the supra-epicondylar region of the femur and arches forward within the deeper substance of the ITB toward its insertion lateral to the Gerdy tubercle.[24,25] This insertion is in a similar location to the ALL, and may also contribute to the Segond fracture.[26] Based on their anatomic observations, Vieira and colleagues[25] suggested that because of the previously described attachments, the "capsulo-osseous layer" of the ITB tended to be stretched with knee in extension, which when combined with the coronal orientation of its fibers, results in a restraint preventing the anterolateral subluxation of the tibia.

Terry and colleagues[27] noted that the deep ITB had been damaged in 93% of functionally unstable knees that were reconstructed and that this damage correlated significantly with the grade of the pivot shift. Recently, Kittl and colleagues[28] studied the efficacy of the anterolateral structures in controlling rotation and found that at full knee extension, the ACL was a significant restraint in the intact knee; with ACL deficiency, that role fell onto the deep layer of the ITB and that neither the ALL nor anterolateral capsular structures offered significant resistance to tibial internal rotation from 0° to 90° of flexion (**Fig. 1**).

In summary, the anterolateral soft tissues contribute to rotational stability in ACL-deficient knees, with the deep ITB possibly playing a more important role closer to extension compared with the ALL, with increasing control of internal rotation in higher-flexion angles.

LATERAL EXTRA-ARTICULAR TENODESIS

The extra-articular procedures and subsequent modifications aimed at restraining anterior translation and rotation in ACL-deficient knees, before the era of arthroscopic ACL reconstruction, are numerous and inherently nonanatomic in design. Some of the more popular techniques of the era are the Lemaire[29] technique, modified Lemaire procedure,[30] Losee[31] technique, MacIntosh "lateral substitution reconstruction,"[32] and Ellison distal iliotibial tract transfer. Most of the techniques used a strip of the

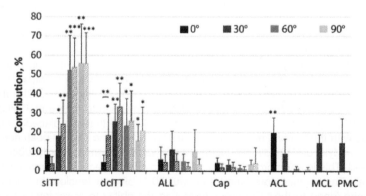

Fig. 1. The contribution of several structures of the knee in controlling 5 Nm of internal rotation torque at varying flexion angles. Cap, anterolateral capsule; dcITT, deep + capsule-osseous iliotibial tract; MCL, medial collateral ligament; PMC, posteromedial corner; sITT, superficial iliotibial tract. (*From* Kittl C, El-Daou H, Athwal KK, et al. The role of the anterolateral structures and the ACL in controlling laxity of the intact and ACL-deficient knee. Am J Sports Med 2016;44 (2):350; with permission.)

ITB with variable length that was tunneled either over or under the FCL and anchored at differing points at the lateral femoral condyle.

Results for the various LET procedures, when done in isolation, have been generally poor.[33,34] Return to previous level of sport was seen in fewer than half of the patients with a MacIntosh procedure, despite a negative pivot shift in 84% of patients.[32] The techniques were noted to result in lateral overconstraint, abnormal resting tibial position in external rotation, and subsequent development of osteoarthritis.[35-37] This has been attributed to tensioning the LET grafts in excessive external rotation, especially in cases in which LET was used as the sole means of compensating for ACL insufficiency. Although overconstraint has the theoretic potential of increasing the lateral compartment reaction forces and hence the risk of osteoarthritis,[38] currently there is little evidence of increased lateral compartment degenerative change in the literature, when LET is combined with ACL reconstruction. A recent systematic review by Hewison and colleagues[39] showed that the addition of an LET to a single-bundle ACL reconstruction resulted in a statistically significant reduction in pivot shift postoperatively (**Fig. 2**) with no difference noted in the rate of osteoarthritis among the studies included.

BIOMECHANICAL STUDIES OF ANTEROLATERAL RECONSTRUCTIONS

Spencer and colleagues[40] investigated both sectioning and reconstruction of the ALL using navigation and manually applied forces. They measured an increase in internal rotation in extension of 2° after division of the ALL in the ACL-deficient knee while performing a simulated pivot shift. Reconstruction of the ALL did not restore the kinematics of the native ALL intact state. However, an LET performed using a strip of the ITB routed under the FCL, and attached to the distal femoral metaphysis (modified Lemaire technique) resulted in a significant reduction in anterior translation and internal rotation in the ACL-deficient state. They postulated that because the LET was routed under the FCL, the latter structure acted as a pulley maintaining relative isometry, whereas the ALL with a distal and anterior origin was lax approaching extension and unlikely to be effective in controlling the pivot shift. They noticed the tendency of an ALL reconstruction to overconstrain the lateral compartment, which is a concern that has been raised from the study of Schon and colleagues[41] as well. The latter authors had concluded that none of the currently recommended anatomic ALL graft fixation angles reported in the literature were capable of restoring anterolateral stability without introducing significant overconstraint of the knee.

Inderhaug and colleagues[42] in a cadaver model using a 6° of freedom rig and an optical tracking system compared 2 different lateral tenodeses (the modified Lemaire technique with graft passed deep to the lateral collateral ligament [LCL] and the MacIntosh tenodesis) with an ALL reconstruction, tensioned to 40 N and 20 N of tension at fixation. The ALL reconstruction used a gracilis graft that was placed superficial to the LCL with the femoral attachment located proximal and slightly posterior to the lateral epicondyle, and the distal attachment midway between the Gerdy tubercle and fibular head. This is a femoral attachment in keeping with recent ALL reconstruction techniques. The investigators found that with 20 N of graft tension, the MacIntosh and Lemaire (deep to the FCL) procedures had the ability to resist internal rotation similar to the intact knee, whereas the ALL reconstruction did not restore native knee kinematics and had persisting increased rotation as compared with the intact knee. The Lemaire superficial procedure (in which the graft was passed over the FCL), provided the least favorable kinematic effects, leading the investigators to infer that the "pulley effect" of the LCL, retaining the graft posterior to the axis of rotation

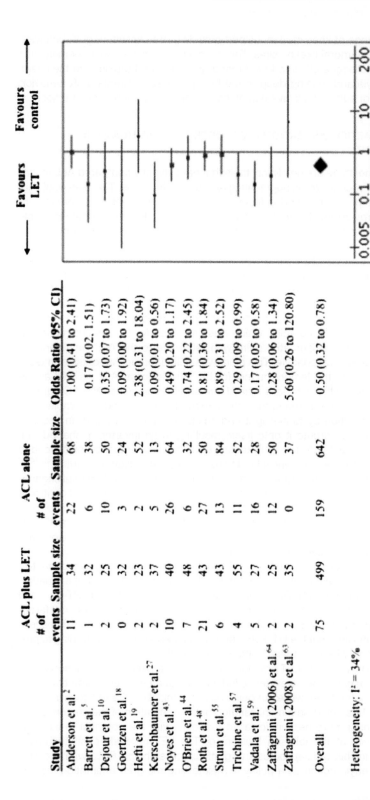

Fig. 2. Forrest plot of pivot shift meta-analyses comparing ACL reconstruction alone versus ACL reconstruction augmented with LET. (*From* Hewison CE, Tran MN, Kaniki N, et al. Lateral extra-articular tenodesis reduces rotational laxity when combined with anterior cruciate ligament reconstruction: a systematic review of the literature. Arthroscopy 2015;31(10):2029; with permission.)

throughout the range of knee motion, helped provide more consistent graft behavior, even with differing femoral fixation sites. This conclusion of theirs is in agreement with that of Kittl and colleagues,[19] who found that a graft attached proximal to the lateral femoral epicondyle and running deep to the FCL provided desirable graft behavior, such that it did not suffer excessive tightening or slackening during knee motion.

LATERAL EXTRA-ARTICULAR TENODESIS OR ANTEROLATERAL LIGAMENT RECONSTRUCTION?

At this point in time, there are no clinical trials that have directly compared ALL reconstruction with LET procedures in augmenting ACL reconstructions. The inferences that can be made are preliminary and indirect based on experimental data from in vitro studies, which provide results at "time zero" and do not take into account possible changes due to healing or graft response to cyclic loading and rehabilitation.

Several techniques have recently been described for anatomic ALL reconstruction based on currently recognized ALL attachment points.[16,43–47] The ALL reconstruction technique with the largest available published clinical data is that of Sonnery-Cottet and colleagues.[46] They described a combined ACL with ALL reconstruction technique that used a 3-strand semitendinosus graft coupled to a free gracilis tendon graft, resulting in a graft that hence had a quadrupled section, used for ACL reconstruction, tailing into a single strand of gracilis, which was then used for ALL reconstruction. In their technique, a femoral isometric point with reference to the ALL was identified close to the lateral femoral condyle. This point was drilled through an outside-in technique to serve both as the femoral tunnel for the intra-articular ACL as well as the femoral attachment for the extra-articular ALL reconstruction. Once the ACL graft is tunneled, the gracilis strand exiting from the femoral tunnel is used to complete the distal ALL reconstruction by tunneling it underneath the ITB and using an osseous tibial tunnel distally to reroute it onto itself, resulting in an inverted Y-shaped ALL reconstruction. This distal double-limb technique differs from most other described ALL reconstruction techniques, which tend to use a single tibial fixation point.[16,43,44,47] It is possible that the 2 bundles spread apart at the tibia provide for differential engagement of individual bundles, resulting in net isometricity and better rotational control at varying flexion angles, making it a biomechanically different construct compared with a single-bundle ALL reconstruction. That being said, the appearance of the graft does also mimic a lateral tenodesis and as such may behave in a similar manner. However, this possibility does not seem to have been tested yet.

Recently Sonnery-Cottet and colleagues[48] published their results of a prospective cohort study of 502 patients. They had stratified their patients into 3 groups: quadrupled hamstring tendon (4HT), bone patellar tendon bone (B-PT-B), and hamstring + ALL graft (HT + ALL). In their study, they found that the rate of graft failure with HT + ALL grafts was 2.5 times less than with B-PT-B grafts and 3.1 times less than with 4HT grafts and that the HT + ALL group had greater odds of returning to pre-injury levels of sport when compared with the 4HT graft.

Our preference is to use the LET procedure rather than an ALL reconstruction where indicated. This is because of the evidence indicating that an ALL reconstruction could overconstrain the lateral joint while not being as mechanically advantageous in resisting rotation.[40–42] This could be a manifestation of the orientation of the anatomic ALL reconstruction being more perpendicular to the joint, with the potential to increase compressive forces at the joint on tensioning. The LET reconstruction technique (described later in this article) routes the graft underneath the FCL, with the FCL and lateral epicondyle acting as a pulley in maintaining the graft orientation more in line with the joint for most of the flexion range. This may help in maintaining the graft at a relatively isometric position and also in a mechanically advantageous vector (to resist rotation), compared with a graft oriented more perpendicular to the joint. Although LET is a nonanatomic reconstruction, it could have the theoretic effect of recruiting more fibers of the ITB into an orientation similar to that of the capsulo-osseous layer of the ITB, but in a deeper plane.

INDICATIONS

At this point in time, there is no clear evidence for the indications for use of an LET in the primary ACL reconstruction setting. In the absence of set criteria, an additional procedure could be a consideration in patient groups known to be at an increased risk of reinjury and graft failure including the following:

- Young age[49,50]
- Patients returning to contact pivoting sport (soccer, rugby, alpine skiing)[49,51]
- Excessive posterior tibial slope of greater than 12°[52]
- Meniscal deficiency[53]

A high-grade pivot shift preoperatively (grade 2 or 3) without a meniscal or collateral ligament injury has been proposed as an indication for consideration of an LET procedure.[54] This type of abnormal pivot shift can be the result of permanent capsular strain, generalized ligamentous laxity, or underlying bony morphologic abnormalities in the lateral compartment.

In the context of revision ACL reconstruction with no coexisting pathology (postero-lateral corner, medial collateral ligament repair, meniscus transplantation), the addition of an extra-articular tenodesis is used. This is supported by the study of Trojani and colleagues,[55] in which a negative pivot shift was found in 80% of ACL revision surgeries combined with an LET in comparison to 63% in ACL revision reconstruction alone.

We are currently performing a randomized clinical trial at our institution (clinicaltrials. gov NCT02018354) comparing ACL reconstruction with or without LET augmentation in patients who are deemed at high risk of graft failure. In time, we hope to be able to further define the ideal indications for the addition of an LET to primary ACL reconstruction.

PREFERRED TECHNIQUE

We use a modified Lemaire procedure with graft passage deep to the FCL as our ante-rolateral augmentation technique, for the reasons explained previously (**Fig. 3**).

A 6-cm curvilinear incision is made just posterior to the lateral femoral epicondyle. The dissection is continued until the posterior border of the ITB has been identified, with any fascial attachments being removed until the level of the Gerdy tubercle. A strip of ITB 1-cm wide and 8-cm in length is dissected from the anterior aspect of the posterior half of the ITB after identifying the location of the capsule-osseous layer of the ITB. We ensure that the capsulo-osseous layer of the deep ITB fibers are not violated. The insertion of the ITB strip at the Gerdy tubercle also remains intact, with any deep attachments of the strip to vastus lateralis removed. Subsequently, the ITB graft is released proximally and a #1 Vicryl whip stitch is placed in the free end of the graft. The FCL is then identified, facilitated by placing the leg in the figure-of-4 position, which places the ligament under tension. Once the FCL has been identified, small capsular incisions are made anterior and posterior to the proximal portion of the ligament and Metzenbaum scissors are placed deep to the FCL to bluntly dissect out a tract for graft passage. One must try to remain extracapsular, ensuring no iatrogenic damage to the

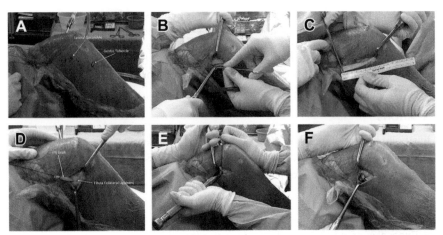

Fig. 3. Surgical technique of the modified Lemaire LET. (*A*) A 6-cm curvilinear incision (*dotted line*) is placed just posterior to the lateral femoral epicondyle. (*B, C*) An 8-cm long × 1-cm wide strip of ITB is harvested from the posterior half of the ITB, ensuring that the most posterior fibers of the capsulo-osseous layer remain intact. (*D*) The FCL is identified and the ITB graft is then passed beneath the FCL from distal to proximal. (*E*) The attachment site should be identified just anterior and proximal to the lateral gastrocnemius tendon. The graft is fixed with a small Richards staple, held taught but not overtensioned, with the knee at 60° flexion and the foot in neutral rotation to avoid lateral compartment overconstraint. (*F*) The graft is sutured back on itself and the ITB is left open to avoid overtightening the lateral retinaculum.

popliteus tendon. The ITB graft is then guided under the FCL from distal to proximal. By using electro cautery, a small fat pad found proximal to the lateral head of gastrocnemius is removed, clearing the lateral femoral supracondylar area exposing the femoral fixation site of the ITB strip, which is located just anterior and proximal to the lateral gastrocnemius tendon. The periosteum is removed by using a cob on the metaphyseal flare of the lateral femoral condyle. The graft is then held taught but not overtensioned, with the knee at 60° flexion and the foot in neutral rotation to avoid lateral compartment overconstraint. The graft is fixated by a small Richards staple (Smith and Nephew, Inc, Andover, MA) and then looped back distally and sutured to itself using the #1 Vicryl whip stitch. The wound is irrigated, hemostasis is confirmed, and closure is performed in layers. We do not close the ITB defect where the graft was harvested from at the level of the transverse ligament to avoid overtightening the lateral patellofemoral joint. However, the defect is reapproximated at the level of vastus lateralis. Weight bearing and range of motion is allowed as tolerated immediately, with the ACL reconstruction and meniscal pathology dictating rehabilitation.

SUMMARY

The soft tissue stabilizers at the anterolateral corner of the knee may offer a solution to minimize the risk of persistent pivot shift in subsets of patients with ACL reconstruction. Our preferred augmentation technique is a LET, for reasons cited previously. The clinical and experimental evidence on the topic has been increasing over the past decade; however, a consensus regarding the long-term clinical efficacy and indications of the procedure has not been reached at this point in time. We are currently undertaking a multicenter randomized controlled trial in an effort to answer these key questions.

REFERENCES

1. Kocher MS, Steadman JR, Briggs KK, et al. Relationships between objective assessment of ligament stability and subjective assessment of symptoms and function after anterior cruciate ligament reconstruction. Am J Sports Med 2004; 32(3):629–34.
2. Ayeni OR, Chahal M, Tran MN, et al. Pivot shift as an outcome measure for ACL reconstruction: a systematic review. Knee Surg 2012;20(4):767–77.
3. Andriacchi TP, Briant PL, Bevill SL, et al. Rotational changes at the knee after ACL injury cause cartilage thinning. Clin Orthop Relat Res 2006;442:39–44.
4. Zampeli F, Ntoulia A, Giotis D, et al. Correlation between anterior cruciate ligament graft obliquity and tibial rotation during dynamic pivoting activities in patients with anatomic anterior cruciate ligament reconstruction: an in vivo examination. Arthroscopy 2012;28(2):234–46.
5. Webster KE, Wotherspoon S, Feller JA, et al. The effect of anterior cruciate ligament graft orientation on rotational knee kinematics. Knee Surg Sports Traumatol Arthrosc 2013;21(9):2113–20.
6. Porter MD, Shadbolt B. Anatomic" single-bundle anterior cruciate ligament reconstruction reduces both anterior translation and internal rotation during the pivot shift. Am J Sports Med 2014;42(12):2948–54.
7. Debandi A, Maeyama A, Hoshino Y, et al. The effect of tunnel placement on rotational stability after ACL reconstruction: evaluation with use of triaxial accelerometry in a porcine model. Knee Surg Sports Traumatol Arthrosc 2013;21(3):589–95.
8. Desai N, Alentorn-Geli E, van Eck CF, et al. A systematic review of single- versus double-bundle ACL reconstruction using the anatomic anterior cruciate ligament reconstruction scoring checklist. Knee Surg Sports Traumatol Arthrosc 2016; 24(3):862–72.
9. Ferretti A, Monaco E, Labianca L, et al. Double-bundle anterior cruciate ligament reconstruction: a computer-assisted orthopaedic surgery study. Am J Sports Med 2008;36(4):760–6.
10. Monaco E, Ferretti A, Labianca L, et al. Navigated knee kinematics after cutting of the ACL and its secondary restraint. Knee Surg Sports Traumatol Arthrosc 2012; 20(5):870–7.
11. Ségond P. Recherches Cliniques Et Expérimentales Sur Les Épanchements Sanguins Du Genou Par Entorse. Progčs Médicale; 1879. p. 297–341.
12. Hughston JC, Andrews JR, Cross MJ, et al. Classification of knee ligament instabilities. Part II. The lateral compartment. J Bone Joint Surg Am 1976;58(2):173–9.
13. Claes S, Luyckx T, Vereecke E, et al. The Segond fracture: a bony injury of the anterolateral ligament of the knee. Arthroscopy 2014;30(11):1475–82.
14. Van Dyck P, Clockaerts S, Vanhoenacker FM, et al. Anterolateral ligament abnormalities in patients with acute anterior cruciate ligament rupture are associated with lateral meniscal and osseous injuries. Eur Radiol 2016;26(10):3383–91.
15. Caterine S, Litchfield R, Johnson M, et al. A cadaveric study of the anterolateral ligament: re-introducing the lateral capsular ligament. Knee Surg Sports Traumatol Arthrosc 2015;23(11):3186–95.
16. Claes S, Vereecke E, Maes M, et al. Anatomy of the anterolateral ligament of the knee. J Anat 2013;223(4):321–8.
17. Kennedy MI, Claes S, Fuso FA, et al. The anterolateral ligament: an anatomic, radiographic, and biomechanical analysis. Am J Sports Med 2015;43(7): 1606–15.

18. Dodds AL, Halewood C, Gupte CM, et al. The anterolateral ligament: anatomy, length changes and association with the Segond fracture. Bone Joint J 2014; 96B(3):325–31.

19. Kittl C, Halewood C, Stephen JM, et al. Length change patterns in the lateral extra-articular structures of the knee and related reconstructions. Am J Sports Med 2015;43(2):354–62.

20. Krackow KA, Brooks RL. Optimization of knee ligament position for lateral extra-articular reconstruction. Am J Sports Med 1983;11(5):293–302.

21. Parsons EM, Gee AO, Spiekerman C, et al. The biomechanical function of the anterolateral ligament of the knee. Am J Sports Med 2015;43(3):669–74.

22. Zantop T, Herbort M, Raschke MJ, et al. The role of the anteromedial and posterolateral bundles of the anterior cruciate ligament in anterior tibial translation and internal rotation. Am J Sports Med 2007;35(2):223–7.

23. Kaplan EB. The iliotibial tract; clinical and morphological significance. J Bone Joint Surg Am 1958;40A(4):817–32.

24. Terry GC, Hughston JC, Norwood LA. The anatomy of the iliopatellar band and iliotibial tract. Am J Sports Med 1986;14(1):39–45.

25. Vieira EL, Vieira EA, da Silva RT, et al. An anatomic study of the iliotibial tract. Arthroscopy 2007;23(3):269–74.

26. Terry GC, LaPrade RF. The biceps femoris muscle complex at the knee. Its anatomy and injury patterns associated with acute anterolateral-anteromedial rotatory instability. Am J Sports Med 1996;24(1):2–8.

27. Terry GC, Norwood LA, Hughston JC, et al. How iliotibial tract injuries of the knee combine with acute anterior cruciate ligament tears to influence abnormal anterior tibial displacement. Am J Sports Med 1993;21(1):55–60.

28. Kittl C, El-Daou H, Athwal KK, et al. The role of the anterolateral structures and the ACL in controlling laxity of the intact and ACL-deficient knee. Am J Sports Med 2016;44(2):345–54.

29. Lemaire M. Ruptures anciennes du ligament croise anterieur du genou. J Chir 1967;(93):311–20.

30. Christel P, Djian P. Anterio-lateral extra-articular tenodesis of the knee using a short strip of fascia lata. Rev Chir Orthop Reparatrice Appar Mot 2002;88(5): 508–13 [in French].

31. Losee RE, Johnson TR, Southwick WO. Anterior subluxation of the lateral tibial plateau. A diagnostic test and operative repair. J Bone Joint Surg Am 1978; 60(8):1015–30.

32. Ireland J, Trickey EL. Macintosh tenodesis for anterolateral instability of the knee. Bone Joint J 1980;62(3):340–5.

33. Fox JM, Blazina ME, Del Pizzo W, et al. Extra-articular stabilization of the knee joint for anterior instability. Clin Orthop Relat Res 1980;(147):56–61.

34. Neyret P, Palomo JR, Donell ST, et al. Extra-articular tenodesis for anterior cruciate ligament rupture in amateur skiers. Br J Sports Med 1994;28(1):31–4.

35. Amis AA, Scammell BE. Biomechanics of intra-articular and extra-articular reconstruction of the anterior cruciate ligament. Bone Joint J 1993;75(5):812–7.

36. Draganich LF, Reider B, Miller PR. An in vitro study of the Müller anterolateral femorotibial ligament tenodesis in the anterior cruciate ligament deficient knee. Am J Sports Med 1989;17(3):357–62.

37. Engebretsen L, Lew WD, Lewis JL, et al. The effect of an iliotibial tenodesis on intraarticular graft forces and knee joint motion. Am J Sports Med 1990;18(2): 169–76.

38. Strum GM, Fox JM, Ferkel RD, et al. Intraarticular versus intraarticular and extra-articular reconstruction for chronic anterior cruciate ligament instability. Clin Orthop Relat Res 1989;(245):188–98.

39. Hewison CE, Tran MN, Kaniki N, et al. Lateral extra-articular tenodesis reduces rotational laxity when combined with anterior cruciate ligament reconstruction: a systematic review of the literature. Arthroscopy 2015;31(10):2022–34.

40. Spencer L, Burkhart TA, Tran MN, et al. Biomechanical analysis of simulated clinical testing and reconstruction of the anterolateral ligament of the knee. Am J Sports Med 2015;43(9):2189–97.

41. Schon JM, Moatshe G, Brady AW, et al. Anatomic anterolateral ligament reconstruction of the knee leads to overconstraint at any fixation angle. Am J Sports Med 2016;44(10):2546–56.

42. Inderhaug E, Stephen JM, Williams A, et al. Biomechanical comparison of anterolateral procedures combined with anterior cruciate ligament reconstruction. Am J Sports Med 2017;45(2):347–54.

43. Colombet P. Knee laxity control in revision anterior cruciate ligament reconstruction versus anterior cruciate ligament reconstruction and lateral tenodesis: clinical assessment using computer-assisted navigation. Am J Sports Med 2011;39(6): 1248–54.

44. Smith JO, Yasen SK, Lord B, et al. Combined anterolateral ligament and anatomic anterior cruciate ligament reconstruction of the knee. Knee Surg Sports Traumatol Arthrosc 2015;23(11):3151–6.

45. Helito CP, Bonadio MB, Gobbi RG, et al. Combined intra- and extra-articular reconstruction of the anterior cruciate ligament: the reconstruction of the knee anterolateral ligament. Arthrosc Tech 2015;4(3):e239–44.

46. Sonnery-Cottet B, Thaunat M, Freychet B, et al. Outcome of a combined anterior cruciate ligament and anterolateral ligament reconstruction technique with a minimum 2-year follow-up. Am J Sports Med 2015;43(7):1598–605.

47. Chahla J, Menge TJ, Mitchell JJ, et al. Anterolateral ligament reconstruction technique: an anatomic-based approach. Arthrosc Tech 2016;5(3):e453–7.

48. Sonnery-Cottet B, Saithna A, Cavalier M, et al. Anterolateral ligament reconstruction is associated with significantly reduced ACL graft rupture rates at a minimum follow-up of 2 years. Am J Sports Med 2017;45(7):1547–57.

49. Kaeding CC, Pedroza AD, Reinke EK, et al, MOON Consortium. Risk factors and predictors of subsequent ACL injury in either knee after ACL reconstruction: prospective analysis of 2488 primary ACL reconstructions from the MOON cohort. Am J Sports Med 2015;43(7):1583–90.

50. Webster KE, Feller JA. Exploring the high reinjury rate in younger patients undergoing anterior cruciate ligament reconstruction. Am J Sports Med 2016;44(11): 2827–32.

51. Agel J, Rockwood T, Klossner D. Collegiate ACL injury rates across 15 sports: National Collegiate Athletic Association Injury Surveillance System data update (2004-2005 through 2012-2013). Clin J Sport Med 2016;26(6):518–23.

52. Rahnemai-Azar AA, Yaseen Z, van Eck CF, et al. Increased lateral tibial plateau slope predisposes male college football players to anterior cruciate ligament injury. J Bone Joint Surg Am 2016;98(12):1001–6.

53. Robb C, Kempshall P, Getgood A, et al. Meniscal integrity predicts laxity of anterior cruciate ligament reconstruction. Knee Surg Sports Traumatol Arthrosc 2015; 23(12):3683–90.

54. Musahl V, Kopf S, Rabuck S, et al. Rotatory knee laxity tests and the pivot shift as tools for ACL treatment algorithm. Knee Surg Sports Traumatol Arthrosc 2012; 20(4):793–800.

55. Trojani C, Beaufils P, Burdin G, et al. Revision ACL reconstruction: influence of a lateral tenodesis. Knee Surg Sports Traumatol Arthrosc 2012;20(8): 1565–70.

Extra-Articular Tenodesis in Combination with Anterior Cruciate Ligament Reconstruction: An Overview

Simone Cerciello, MD[a,b,*], Cécile Batailler, MD[c],
Nader Darwich, MD[d], Philippe Neyret, MD, PhD[d]

KEYWORDS

- Anterior cruciate ligament • Extra-articular tenodesis • Pivot shift • Graft failure
- Anterolateral ligament

KEY POINTS

- Anterior cruciate ligament (ACL) reconstruction is a successful operation; however, persistent instability is sometimes reported.
- The anterolateral structures of the knee, including the recently described anterolateral ligament, have an important role in the control of the pivot shift phenomenon.
- The results of isolated reconstruction of the anterolateral structures in the ACL deficient knees are poor in terms of stability and patient satisfaction.
- Combined ACL reconstruction and anterolateral ligament reconstruction or lateral extra-articular tenodesis procedures increase knee stability and may reduce the failure rate of ACL reconstruction in high-demand athletes and in presence of a high-grade pivot shift.

INTRODUCTION

Anterior cruciate ligament (ACL) injuries are common, with an overall reported incidence of 68.6 cases per 100,000 population per year.[1] The role of the ACL in knee stability has been widely demonstrated. Rotatory stability is essential and is achieved through the interaction between ACL and peripheral structures. Surgical reconstruction of a torn ACL is indicated to restore knee stability, to prevent secondary injuries

Disclosure Statement: The authors declare that they have no direct financial interest in subject matter or materials discussed in article.
[a] Orthopaedic Surgery, Casa di Cura Villa Betania, Via Piccolomini 27, Rome 00165, Italy;
[b] Orthopaedic Surgery, Marrelli Hospital, Via Gioacchino da Fiore, Crotone 0962, Italy;
[c] Orthopaedic Surgery, Albert Trillat Center, Lyon North University Hospital, 103 Grande Rue de la Croix-Rousse, Lyon 69004, France; [d] Healthpoint, Abu Dhabi Knee & Sports Medicine Center, Zayed Sports City, Abu Dhabi, United Arab Emirates
* Corresponding author. Orthopaedic Surgery, Casa di Cura Villa Betania, Via Piccolomini 27, Rome 00165, Italy.
E-mail address: simone.cerciello@me.com

Clin Sports Med 37 (2018) 87–100
http://dx.doi.org/10.1016/j.csm.2017.07.006
0278-5919/18/© 2017 Elsevier Inc. All rights reserved.

to menisci and cartilage, and to ideally prevent the development of osteoarthritis (OA).[2] The outcomes with all modern surgical techniques are extremely positive, with 90% of patients reporting normal or nearly normal knee function, 82% returning to sports participation, 63% regaining their preinjury level of participation, and 44% returning to competitive sport at final follow-up.[3] Despite this success, residual rotatory instability persists in 11% to 30% of patients.[4–6]

Rotatory instability has been observed even following successful reconstruction and is among the most critical aspects in patient satisfaction. Compared with the transtibial technique, reconstruction of the ACL through an anatomic single-bundle procedure has the advantage of improved rotatory stability.[7–9] However, such reconstructions subject the graft to higher stresses, increasing failure rates.[10] More recently, the double-bundle technique has been proposed, but unfortunately there is no clear evidence of better control of rotational laxity.[11–13] Two meta-analyses showed that up to 34% of patients after single-bundle and 22% of patients after double-bundle reconstruction continue to have a positive pivot shift.[14,15] Rotational instability has been related to multiple factors, including increased tibial slope and injury to the lateral meniscus, posterolateral corner, and more recently, the anterolateral ligament (ALL).[16–19]

Ségond first showed the involvement of lateral structures after ACL injuries, reporting an avulsion fracture of the proximal tibia.[20] Almost 100 years later, Norwood and colleagues[21] analyzed a series of 36 patients with anterolateral rotatory instability. Isolated ACL injury was present only in 4 patients, while concomitant injury to the lateral structures (from lateral capsule to iliotibial tract) was observed in 26 patients. Several authors have identified and described a structure connecting the lateral femoral condyle, lateral meniscus, and lateral tibial plateau.[22–25] In the literature, it has been described as the capsulo-osseous layer of the iliotibial tract, midthird lateral capsular ligament, lateral capsular ligament, or ALL. Accordingly, techniques have been developed to repair/reconstruct the injured structures of the anterolateral aspect of the knee in association with an ACL reconstruction.

ANATOMY AND BIOMECHANICS

Ségond was the first to describe a "pearly, resistant, fibrous band which invariably showed extreme amounts of tension during forced internal rotation."[20] This can be considered the first description of the ALL. The ALL originates as a complex of fan-like blending fibers[26] from the prominence of the lateral femoral epicondyle, anterior to the origin of the LCL and just proximal and posterior to the insertion of the popliteus tendon, inserting between the Gerdy tubercle and the fibular head.[18,27] Most fibers merge with the lateral meniscus[19]; however, Claes and colleagues[18] described meniscotibial and meniscofemoral bundles. This ALL has a dense, regularly organized structure with additional peripheral nervous innervation and mechanoreceptors.[28–32] Hughston and colleagues found that sectioning the lateral capsular ligament resulted in a major increase of anterolateral rotatory instability.[33] Monaco and colleagues,[34] in a study on 10 fresh-frozen specimens, evaluated the anterior tibial translation (ATT) and internal rotation (IR) in intact knees and after selectively transecting both the ACL anteromedial bundle (AM) and posterolateral bundle (PL), and then the ALL. A significant increase in ATT at 60° and IR at 30°, 45°, and 60° was found after ALL sectioning, supporting the conclusion that concomitant injury to the ALL is related to the pivot shift phenomenon. A more recent study by Parsons and colleagues[35] confirmed that the ALL is an important stabilizer of internal rotation at flexion angles greater than 35°, while the ACL is the primary restraint to ATT at all flexion angles and to IR at flexion angles less than 35°. Claes and colleagues,[36] in a retrospective review of 271 MRI studies in patients with ACL injury, found the ALL to be clearly visible in 206 patients and torn in 162 (78.8%) patients. An associated bony avulsion (Ségond fracture) was noted in 1.8% of patients.

The ALL is not the only part of the anterolateral complex to play a role in knee stability. Posterior root tears and overall deficiency of the lateral meniscus can also contribute to rotatory instability in ACL-deficient knees.[37,38] Furthermore, the capsule-osseous layer of the iliotibial band (ITB), running proximally from the posterior Kaplan fibers on the distal femur to the posterior aspect of the Gerdy tubercle, also plays a major role in rotatory stability.[39]

INDICATIONS AND RATIONALE FOR LATERAL EXTRA-ARTICULAR TENODESIS

Extra-articular tenodesis (EAT) techniques were initially performed as isolated procedures; however, they were criticized due to poor control of anterior tibial translation.[40] Failure rates greater than 50% have been reported in athletes, especially in cases with associated medial meniscus tears.[41] As a result, isolated extra-articular procedures are no longer recommended.[41] Studies have shown that combined procedures may be more beneficial. Extra-articular lateral tenodesis has been shown to decrease loads on the ACL graft by 43%, which may reduce the risk of repeat rupture.[42,43] EAT has also been shown to increase stability in patients with combined ACL and anterolateral capsular deficiencies.[44] EAT is contraindicated in the presence of a posterolateral corner injury.[45] In these cases, the tenodesis may tether the tibia in a subluxed position, posterolaterally. To date, there is no clear consensus regarding the clinical indications for a combined ACL reconstruction and EAT. A recent systematic review showed that extra-articular procedures were effective in reducing the pivot shift phenomenon and therefore should be considered in patients with a markedly positive pivot shift test.[46] Patients with large amounts of anterior translation in the lateral compartment may also benefit from an EAT.[47] Additionally, it should be considered in patients who play contact sports or who are undergoing revision ACL reconstruction. In these cases, the addition of an EAT may increase stability and reduce the failure rate.[48,49] Specifically, combined ACL reconstruction and EAT should be considered:

- In patients with major (3+) pivot shift test and healthy medial meniscus and medial collateral ligament[50]
- In young patients (age <25 years)
- In cases of genu recurvatum greater than 10°
- In patients playing contact sports
- In patients with generalized ligamentous laxity
- In cases of revision ACL reconstruction without a clear reason for failure

It can also be considered in patients with high risk of re-rupture, such as adolescent female soccer players or when a large medial meniscectomy is performed.[51–53]

ISOLATED EXTRA-ARTICULAR TENODESIS

The techniques for isolated EAT described were initially introduced as isolated procedures; however, they can be performed in combination with ACL reconstruction.

Lemaire Procedure

A strip of the ITB measuring 18 cm in length and 1 to 1.5 cm in width, inserted on the Gerdy tubercle, is harvested. Two osseous tunnels are then prepared; the femoral tunnel is located just above the lateral epicondyle and proximal to the LCL, while the tibial tunnel is made through the Gerdy tubercle.[54] The graft is then passed under the LCL (**Fig. 1**), through the femoral bone tunnel, back under the LCL, finally inserting into the Gerdy tubercle via the tibial tunnel. Tensioning and fixation of the graft are performed at 30° of flexion and neutral rotation.

Christel and Dijan described a variation of the Lemaire procedure, which reduces the skin incision length and degree of soft tissue dissection.[55] A graft measuring 75 mm long and 12 mm wide is again mobilized from the Gerdy tubercle. A femoral tunnel is drilled in the isometric point on the lateral femoral condyle (determined by a compass). The graft is not passed under the LCL to avoid devascularization of the LCL. Draganich and colleagues[43] also showed more homogenous graft forces and better isometry when the graft was twisted 180° and fixed with an interference screw.

Ellison Procedure

An osteotome is used to elevate a 1.5 cm button of bone from the Gerdy tubercle.[56] A strip of ITB with a wider proximal end is passed under the LCL. With the knee at 90° of flexion, the graft is fixed with a staple just anterior to the Gerdy tubercle and reinforced with suture. A plication of the midthird capsular ligament can be performed.

MacIntosh Procedure

The technique of lateral substitution is similar to the original Lemaire operation. A strip of the middle third of the ITB approximately 20 cm × 2 cm is harvested, leaving the distal end attached to the Gerdy tubercle.[57] The graft is then passed through a sub-periosteal tunnel behind the origin of the LCL and looped behind the insertion of the lateral intermuscular septum, before passing again under the LCL. With the knee flexed to 90° and the tibia externally rotated, the graft is sutured to the periosteum of the tunnel. After passing the graft deep to the LCL, the ITB strip is looped over the top behind the lateral femoral condyle, through the notch into the joint, and finally secured in a tibial bone tunnel. This variation of the original technique combines an intra- and extra-articular procedure.

Arnold-Coker Procedure

In this modification of the MacIntosh procedure, an ITB strip, measuring 15 to 18 cm × 2 cm, is harvested while preserving the distal insertion on the Gerdy

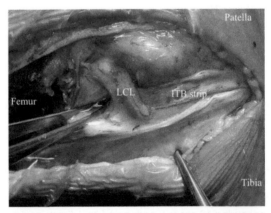

Fig. 1. In the Lemaire procedure, the graft (using forceps) is passed under the LCL and through the femoral bone tunnel before looping back under the LCL toward the Gerdy tubercle.

tubercle.[58] The ITB graft is passed underneath the LCL and brought back to the Gerdy tubercle. The graft is then sutured proximally to the LCL and fixed distally with a staple, keeping the knee at 90° of flexion and external rotation without effort.

Losee Procedure

A 12 to 14 cm × 2.5 cm ITB graft is harvested while preserving its distal insertion.[59] A 9 mm tunnel is drilled at the femoral attachment of the LCL from anterior and inferior to superior and posterior in order to exit at the level of the lateral gastrocnemius tendon. The graft is passed through this tunnel and sutured to the periosteum of both tunnel exits. The graft is then passed back through the lateral gastrocnemius tendon, the posterolateral capsule, posterior to the LCL, and then passed under the LCL itself. The procedure is completed by suturing the ITB graft to the Gerdy tubercle, while the gastrocnemius tendon, the posterolateral capsule, and the graft are all sutured to the LCL (sling and reef effect) with the knee at 45° of flexion.

Andrews Procedure

In 1983, Andrews and Sanders described an extra-articular tenodesis procedure where the ITB is first split for 10 cm in line with its fibers.[60] Both leaflets are then sutured to the lateral aspect of the lateral femur at 30° of flexion and slight external rotation.

Literature Overview

The outcomes of isolated procedures have been generally poor, with persistent instability and low rates of good-to-excellent results (57% to 63% for the Ellison procedure and 52% for the Lemaire procedure).[41,61,62] Neyret and colleagues[41] examined 31 skiers (33 knees) treated with isolated Lemaire procedure. Sixteen patients were satisfied with their functional results, but 9 of 18 patients had positive pivot shift at 1 year, and 12 out 15 patients had positive pivot shift at 4.5 years (final follow-up). Ireland and Trickey reported their results with the MacIntosh procedure in 50 knees at 2-year follow-up.[63] A negative jerk test was reported in 42 of 50 knees (84%), but fewer than 50% of patients were able to return to preinjury level, with less than satisfactory results. Ellison[56] reported good or excellent results in 15 of 18 knees at an average follow-up of 41 months for distal iliotibial band transfer. However, these favorable results[64] have not been uniformly reproduced. Kennedy and colleagues, using the same technique, found that all 28 patients had persistent anterior drawer, and 24 patients had a positive pivot shift at 6 months. These unsatisfactory results are probably a consequence of the nonanatomic reconstruction, which resulted in poor knee kinematics, and insufficient control of tibial translation and rotation.[40] Furthermore, tensioning of the graft in tibial external rotation[40,65,66] may have resulted in progressive stretching of the graft itself and overload of the lateral compartment.[67]

COMBINED EXTRA-ARTICULAR TENODESIS

Early combined procedures used the ITB to augment the anterolateral aspect of the knee.

The Use of the Hamstrings for both Anterior Cruciate Ligament Reconstruction and Lateral Extra-Articular Tenodesis

Marcacci and colleagues[68] described harvesting the gracilis and semitendinosus tendons while leaving their tibial insertions intact. Both tendons are then passed through an 8 to 9 mm tibial tunnel and then over the top of the lateral femoral condyle. Proximal to the lateral epicondyle, a groove is prepared to facilitate graft healing. The graft is fixed into this groove with 2 staples with the knee at 90° of flexion. The remaining graft is then passed deep to the iliotibial band but superficial to the LCL, and secured at the Gerdy tubercle with another staple.

More recently, Colombet[69] described a similar technique. A 21 cm hamstring graft tis prepared after detachment of the tibial insertion. After drilling the femoral and tibial tunnels, an additional tunnel is drilled from the Gerdy tubercle to the hamstring origin. If sufficient graft length is present, a 4-strand intra-articular portion (9 cm) is used to reconstruct the ACL, and a 2-strand extra-articular portion (12 cm) is prepared to perform the lateral tenodesis. In the case of insufficient graft length, both the intra and extra-articular portions can be performed with a 2-strand graft. Fixation is achieved using 2 absorbable interference screws at the level of tibial and femoral tunnel. The extra-articular portion is passed under the ITB but superficial to the LCL, into the Gerdy tubercle tunnel, and finally fixed with an interference screw.

Use of Bone Tendon Bone Autograft for Anterior Cruciate Ligament Reconstruction and the Hamstring Tendons for Lateral Extra-Articular Tenodesis

The ACL reconstruction is performed in an outside-in fashion using a 9 mm central third bone-patellar tendon-bone graft. Both the tibial and femoral tunnels are 10 mm in diameter. The tibial bone block, used on the femoral tunnel, is wider (around 11–12 mm) to host a 4.5 mm drill hole. The femoral tunnel is drilled just posterior and proximal to the origin of the LCL. An additional tunnel is created at the level of the Gerdy tubercle. The gracilis tendon is used for the extra-articular procedure and passed through the tibial bone block hole to obtain 2 strands of the equal length. The patellar tendon graft is introduced into the knee through the femoral tunnel. The tibial bone block is impacted into the tunnel to achieve a press-fit fixation, securing at the same time the gracilis into the bone tunnel. Tibial fixation is achieved with an interference screw. The 2 ends of gracilis are then passed underneath the LCL (**Fig. 2**) and in opposite directions through a bony tunnel created in the Gerdy tubercle. Final fixation is obtained by suturing the ends to each other with the knee held at 30° of flexion.

Mixed Grafts

Marshall and colleagues[70] described a modification of the original MacIntosh procedure to address both the ACL reconstruction and the extra-articular reinforcement. The central third of the entire extensor mechanism was harvested, including part of the

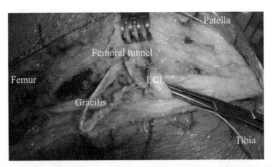

Fig. 2. When performing a combined of ACL reconstruction with Bone Tendon Bone (BTB) autograft and an LET with a gracilis tendon graft, the 2 ends of gracilis tendon are passed underneath the LCL and then through the bony tunnel in the Gerdy tubercle in opposite directions.

prepatellar aponeurotic tissue. The tibial tunnel is drilled at the usual location for ACL reconstruction, and the graft is passed through this tunnel, over the top of the lateral femoral condyle, and fixed to the Gerdy tubercle.

Lerat and colleagues[71] described a combined procedure using the lateral third of the patellar tendon with an attached 10 to 12 cm strip of quadriceps tendon. The tibial tunnel is created in a standard fashion, and the femoral tunnel emerges just proximal to the LCL insertion. An additional tunnel is created at the level of the Gerdy tubercle. The patellar bone graft is shaped to obtain press fit fixation in the femoral tunnel while the tibial bone block is retrieved from the tibial tunnel, tensioned with a metallic wire, and fixed with a 4.5 mm or 3.5 mm metal cortical type screw. With the knee at 60° of flexion, the quadriceps tendon is passed underneath the LCL, through the tunnel, under the Gerdy tubercle, and sutured to itself.

Zarins and Rowe described their technique for combined reconstruction using the ITB and semitendinosus tendon.[72] Both the ITB and semitendinosus grafts are harvested with the distal insertion preserved. Two 25 cm × 2 cm strips are obtained. A 6 mm tibial tunnel is drilled, and an 8 mm groove is made anterior to the over-the-top position. To increase stability, the anterolateral capsule is plicated 1 to 2 cm beneath the LCL. The semitendinosus is passed through the tibial tunnel, retrieved at the over-the-top location, and passed through the femoral groove and then underneath the LCL. The ITB graft has the opposite positioning, passed deep to the lateral collateral ligament, retrieved at the over-the-top location, and passed through the tibial tunnel. Both grafts are tensioned and then fixed with the knee at 60° of flexion, sutured to each other and the underlying posterolateral capsule.

Literature Overview

Combined procedures are successful operations; however, they involve additional large lateral incisions. Persistent pain on the lateral aspect of the knee has been reported in up to 40% of patients.[73] Reports from the 1990s and early 2000s did not show any clear advantage of combined procedures over isolated intra-articular reconstruction.[4,67,73] Recent case series, however, have shown high rates of return to high-impact sports with good control of the pivot shift phenomenon at long-term follow-up.[74–78] In most series, good or excellent results are reported in 80% to 90% of patients.[79] However, when comparing combined and isolated procedures, the increased stability is not always reflected by superior functional outcomes.[48] This has been confirmed in 3 recent systematic reviews and meta-analyses. Rezende and colleagues[80] compared randomized controlled trials (RCT) of isolated ACL reconstruction versus EAT in combination with ACL reconstruction (8 studies). Combined procedures were found to slightly improve knee stability with no clear advantage in terms of failure rates or patient reported outcome scores. A similar meta-analysis by Hewison and colleagues[46] (29 articles, 8 RCTs) revealed a statistically significant reduction of the pivot shift after ACL reconstruction with EAT, but no significant differences in terms of anterior translation or IKDC scores. Song and colleagues,[81] in their systematic review of 7 studies, showed that EAT combined with ACL reconstruction was effective in eliminating the high-grade pivot shift phenomenon, but no differences were reported in terms of objective IKDC score and anterior tibial translation at short-term follow-up when compared with isolated ACL reconstruction.

COMBINED PROCEDURES INVOLVING ANTERO-LATERAL LIGAMENT RECONSTRUCTION

The techniques described are all based on recent anatomic and biomechanical studies of the ALL.

Smith Technique

This technique requires both the semitendinosus and gracilis tendons; the former is used for an all-inside ACL reconstruction, the latter to recreate the ALL.[82] Two 4.5 mm × 25 mm tunnels are created, 1 just anterior and superior to the femoral insertion of the LCL and the second halfway between the Gerdy tubercle and the fibular head, 11 mm below the joint line. A whipstitch is placed in the proximal end of the gracilis tendon, which is then passed into the femoral tunnel and secured with an absorbable, fully threaded, knotless anchor. The graft is then passed underneath the ITB and into the tibial tunnel. Final fixation is performed with another fully threaded knotless anchor with the knee in 30° of flexion.

Helito Technique

This technique requires a tripled semitendinosus and single strand gracilis graft to obtain a 4-stranded ACL and single-stranded ALL.[83] Under fluoroscopic guidance, a 5 mm metal suture anchor is placed at the ALL femoral attachment (3–4 mm distal to the halfway point on the Blumensaat line). The ACL femoral tunnel is made using an outside-in technique, and the tibial tunnel is drilled using a standard ACL drilling guide. The graft is retrieved from distal to proximal to have the 4 strands in the joint. Femoral fixation is performed first, with a bioabsorbable interference screw that is equal to the diameter of the femoral tunnel. Tibial fixation is achieved with bioabsorbable interference screw that is 1 mm greater in size than the tunnel diameter. The knee is held in 30° of flexion and neutral rotation. The gracilis is fixed on the femur using the metal anchor. Tibial fixation is achieved with a second suture anchor positioned at the anatomic insertion off the ALL, halfway between the Gerdy tubercle and the fibular head, 5 to 10 mm below the joint line.[84] The graft is then passed under the ITB and fixed to the second suture anchor at 60° to 90° of flexion.

Sonnery-Cottet Technique

This technique also uses a 4-strand semitendinosus and gracilis hamstring graft with its tibial insertion preserved.[85] The tibial tunnel is performed in a standard fashion. Two stab incisions are then used to create an additional 3.2 mm tunnel connecting the supero-lateral corner of the Gerdy tubercle and the site of the Ségond fracture (more proximal and lateral). The ACL femoral tunnel emerges at the ALL-isometric point. Following fixation of the ACL graft with bioabsorbable screws, the remaining part of the gracilis tendon is passed deep to the ITB but superficial to the LCL, through the ALL tibial tunnel, and then back through the femoral tunnel in order to create a Y-shaped ALL construct. The ALL graft is fixed with an interference screw in extension and neutral rotation and secured at the ACL femoral tunnel with the ACL graft traction sutures.

Wagih Technique

Wagih described a percutaneous technique of ALL reconstruction using polyester tape.[86] A 5 mm transverse skin incision is performed at the level of femoral insertion of the ALL. A 4.5 mm tunnel is drilled over a 2.7 mm passing pin. In a similar way, 2 4.5 mm transverse tunnels are drilled just proximal to the midpoint between the head of the fibula and the Gerdy tubercle, leaving a 1 cm bony bridge. A polyester tape of 4 mm diameter and 60 mm length is loaded over a cortical suspensory fixation button, which is retrieved from the medial femoral tunnel. The 2 free hands of the tape are passed deep to the ITB and retrieved on the lateral aspect of the proximal tibia.

Finally, the 2 strands are passed through the tibial tunnels and tied together over the 1 cm bone bridge with the knee in 30° of flexion.

Literature Overview

Currently there is a paucity of literature regarding outcomes of ALL reconstruction. Sonnery-Cottet and colleagues[6] reported a series of 92 patients with minimum 2-year follow-up who underwent combined ACL and ALL reconstruction. Good or excellent improvement in subjective and objective scores was observed in all patients. A significant pivot shift reduction (grade 0 or grade 1) was also observed in all cases. In another case series by Sonnery-Cottet and colleagues,[87] patients were treated with either combined ACL and ALL reconstruction or isolated ACL reconstruction with Bone Tendon Bone (BTB), or quadruped hamstring. At an average follow-up of 38.4 months, the 221 patients who underwent the combined procedure had a failure rate of 4.13%, which was lower than those who underwent isolated ACL reconstruction irrespective of graft choice. Furthermore, patients who underwent the combined procedure had improved odds of returning to preinjury levels of sport than the isolated ACL reconstruction hamstring group (odds ratio [OR]: 1.938; 95% confidence interval [CI], 1.174–3.224) but not the BTB group (OR: 1.460; 95% CI, 0.813–2.613). Zhang and colleagues[88] reviewed a series of 60 patients treated with either SB ACL reconstruction, DB ACL reconstruction, or combined ACL and ALL reconstruction. At a minimum follow-up of 12 months, the outcomes of DB ACL and combined ACL and ALL were comparable in terms of knee stability and joint function.

SUMMARY

ACL reconstruction is a successful operation with a high patient satisfaction rate and favorable rates for return to sport. Despite this, a subset of patients continue to have persistent rotatory knee instability despite anatomic reconstruction. Recent anatomic and biomechanical studies have highlighted the contribution of peripheral structures such as medial and lateral menisci, ALL, and ITB in controlling tibial rotation. Imaging studies have also reliably demonstrated injury to lateral knee structures when an explosive pivot shift is reported.

Isolated extra-articular procedures result in persistent instability and poor functional outcomes. Combined procedures involving ACL reconstruction and lateral extra-articular tenodesis or ALL reconstruction are effective in reducing the rates of residual instability. Furthermore, the literature supports the biomechanical benefits of providing an extra-articular restraint to internal tibial rotation. Currently, despite ongoing controversy in the orthopedic literature, indications for combined ACL reconstruction and EAT or ALL reconstruction include high grade pivot shift on physical examination, young age, generalized ligamentous laxity, participation in contact sports, and revision surgery without a clear reason for failure. When compared with traditional lateral EAT techniques, modern ALL reconstruction has the advantage of being more anatomic, less invasive, and associated with lower rates of persistent pain on the lateral aspect of the knee.

REFERENCES

1. Sanders TL, MaraditKremers H, Bryan AJ, et al. Incidence of anterior cruciate ligament tears and reconstruction: a 21-year population-based study. Am J Sports Med 2016;44(6):1502–7.

2. Kennedy J, Jackson MP, O'Kelly P, et al. Timing of reconstruction of the anterior cruciate ligament in athletes and the incidence of secondary pathology within the knee. J Bone Joint Surg Br 2010;92:362–6.
3. Ardern CL, Webster KE, Taylor NF, et al. Return to sport following anterior cruciate ligament reconstruction surgery: a systematic review and meta-analysis of the state of play. Br J Sports Med 2011;45:596–606.
4. Anderson AF, Snyder RB, Lipscomb AB Jr. Anterior cruciate ligament reconstruction. A prospective randomized study of three surgical methods. Am J Sports Med 2001;29:272–9.
5. Kocher MS, Steadman JR, Briggs K, et al. Determinants of patient satisfaction with outcome after anterior cruciate ligament reconstruction. J Bone Joint Surg Am 2002;84:1560–72.
6. Sonnery-Cottet B, Thaunat M, Freychet B, et al. Outcome of a combined anterior cruciate ligament and anterolateral ligament reconstruction technique with a minimum 2-year follow-up. Am J Sports Med 2015;43:1598–605.
7. Bedi A, Feeley BT, Williams RJ. Management of articular cartilage defects of the knee. J Bone Joint Surg Am 2010;92:994–1009.
8. Markolf KL, Jackson SR, McAllister DR. A comparison of 11 o'clock versus oblique femoral tunnels in the anterior cruciate ligament reconstructed knee: knee kinematics during a simulated pivot test. Am J Sports Med 2010;38:912–7.
9. Kato Y, Maeyama A, Lertwanich P, et al. Biomechanical comparison of different graft positions for single-bundle anterior cruciate ligament reconstruction. Knee Surg Sports Traumatol Arthrosc 2012;21:816–23.
10. Kato Y, Ingham SJM, Kramer S, et al. Effect of tunnel position for anatomic single-bundle ACL reconstruction on knee biomechanics in a porcine model. Knee Surg Sports Traumatol Arthrosc 2009;18:2–10.
11. Meredick RB, Vance KJ, Appleby D, et al. Outcome of single-bundle versus double-bundle reconstructionof the anterior cruciate ligament: a meta-analysis. Am J Sports Med 2008;36:1414–21.
12. Muneta T, Hara K, Ju YJ, et al. Revision anterior cruciate ligament reconstruction by double-bundle technique using multi-strand semitendinosus tendon. Arthroscopy 2010;26:769–81.
13. Zaffagnini S, Signorelli C, Lopomo N, et al. Anatomic double-bundle and over-the-top single-bundle with additional extra-articulartenodesis: an in vivo quantitative assessment of knee laxity in two different ACL reconstructions. Knee Surg Sports Traumatol Arthrosc 2012;20:153–9.
14. Prodromos CC, Joyce BT, Shi K, et al. A meta-analysis of stability after anterior cruciate ligament reconstruction as a function of hamstring versus patellar tendon graft and fixation type. Arthroscopy 2005;21(10):1202.
15. Mohtadi N. Function after ACL reconstruction: a review. Clin J Sport Med 2008; 18(1):105–6.
16. Matsumoto H, Seedhom BB. Treatment of the pivot-shift intra-articular versus extra-articular or combined reconstruction procedures: a biomechanical study. Clin Orthop Relat Res 1994;299:298–304.
17. Bull AMJ, Amis A. The pivot-shift phenomenon: a clinical and biomechanical perspective. Knee 1998;5(1):141–58.
18. Claes S, Vereecke E, Maes M, et al. Anatomy of the anterolateral ligament of the knee. J Anat 2013;223(4):321–8.
19. Vincent JP, Magnussen RA, Gezmez F, et al. The anterolateral ligament of the human knee: an anatomic and histologic study. Knee Surg Sports Traumatol Arthrosc 2012;20(1):147–52.

20. Ségond P. Recherches cliniques et expérimentales sur les épanchements sanguins du genou par entorse. Prog Med 1879;7:297–9, 319–21, 40–1.
21. Norwood LA, Andrews JR, Meisterling RC, et al. Acute anterolateral rotatory instability of the knee. J Bone Joint Surg Am 1979;61:704–9.
22. Terry GC, Hughston JC, Norwood LA. The anatomy of the iliopatellar band and iliotibial tract. Am J Sports Med 1986;14:39–45.
23. LaPrade RF, Gilbert TJ, Bollom TS, et al. The magnetic resonance imaging appearance of individual structures of the posterolateral knee. A prospective study of normal knees and knees with surgicallyverified grade III injuries. Am J Sports Med 2000;28:191–9.
24. Vieira EL, Vieira EA, Teixeira da Silva R, et al. An anatomic study of the iliotibial tract. Arthroscopy 2007;23:269–74.
25. Irvine GB, Dias JJ, Finlay DB. Segond fractures of the lateral tibial condyle: brief report. J Bone Joint Surg Br 1987;69:613–4.
26. Dodds AL, Halewood C, Gupte CM, et al. The anterolateral ligament: anatomy, length changes and association with the Segond fracture. Bone Joint J 2014; 96:325–31.
27. Kennedy MI, Claes S, Fuso FA, et al. The antero later alligament: An anatomic, radiographic, and biomechanical analysis. Am J Sports Med 2015;43: 431606–15.
28. Caterine S, Litchfield R, Johnson M, et al. A cadaveric study of the anterolateral ligament: re-introducing the lateral capsular ligament. Knee Surg Sports Traumatol Arthrosc 2015;23(11):3186–95.
29. Johnson LL. Lateral capsular ligament complex: anatomical and surgical considerations. Am J Sports Med 1979;7:156–60.
30. Haims AH, Medvecky MJ, Pavlovich R Jr, et al. MR imaging of the anatomy of and injuries to the lateral and posterolateral aspects of the knee. Am J Roentgenol 2003;180:647–53.
31. Moorman CT 3rd, LaPrade RF. Anatomy and biomechanics of the posterolateral corner of the knee. J Knee Surg 2005;18:137–45.
32. Campos JC, Chung CB, Lektrakul N, et al. Pathogenesis of the Segond Fracture: anatomic and MR imaging evidence of an iliotibial tract or anterior oblique band avulsion. Radiology 2001;219:381–6.
33. Hughston JC, Andrews JR, Cross MJ, et al. Classification of knee ligament instabilities. Part II. The lateral compartment. J Bone Joint Surg Am 1976;58:173–9.
34. Monaco E, Ferretti A, Labianca L, et al. Navigated knee kinematics after cutting of the ACL and its secondary restraint. Knee Surg Sports Traumatol Arthrosc 2012; 20:870–7.
35. Parsons EM, Gee AO, Spiekerman C, et al. The biomechanical function of the anterolateral ligament of the knee. Am J Sports Med 2015;43:669–74.
36. Claes S, Bartholomeeusen S, Bellemans J. High prevalence of anterolateral ligament abnormalities in magnetic resonance images of anterior cruciate ligament injured knees. Acta Orthop Belg 2014;80:45–9.
37. Bhatia S, LaPrade CM, Ellman MB, et al. Meniscal root tears: significance, diagnosis, and treatment. Am J Sports Med 2014;42:3016–30.
38. Tanaka M, Vyas D, Moloney G, et al. What does it take to have a high-grade pivot shift? Knee Surg Sports Traumatol Arthrosc 2012;20:737–42.
39. Kittl C, El Daou H, Athwayl K, et al. The role of the anterolateral structures and the ACL in controlling internal rotational knee laxity. Am J Sports Med 2016;44(2): 345–54.

40. Amis AA, Scammell BE. Biomechanics of intra-articular and extra-articular reconstruction of the anterior cruciate ligament. J Bone Joint Surg Br 1993;75:812–7.

41. Neyret P, Palomo JR, Donell ST, et al. Extra-articular tenodesis for anterior cruciate ligament rupture in amateur skiers. Br J Sports Med 1994;28:31–4.

42. Engebretsen L, Lew WD, Lewis JL, et al. The effect of an iliotibial tenodesis on intraarticular graft forces and knee joint motion. Am J Sports Med 1990;18:169–76.

43. Draganich LF, Reider B, Ling M, et al. An in vitro study of an intraarticular and extraarticular reconstruction in the anterior cruciate ligament deficient knee. Am J Sports Med 1990;18:262–6.

44. Samuelson M, Draganich LF, Zhou X, et al. The effects of knee reconstruction on combined anterior cruciate ligament and anterolateral capsular deficiencies. Am J Sports Med 1996;24:492–7.

45. Duthon VB, Magnussen RA, Servien E, et al. ACL reconstruction and extra-articular tenodesis. Clin Sports Med 2013;32:141–53.

46. Hewison CE, Tran MN, Kaniki N, et al. Lateral extra-articular tenodesis reduces rotational laxity when combined with anterior cruciate ligament reconstruction: a systematic review of the literature. Arthroscopy 2015;31(10):2022–34.

47. Lerat JL, Moyen BL, Cladière F, et al. Knee instability after injury to the anterior cruciate ligament. Quantification of the Lachman test. J Bone Joint Surg Br 2000;82:42–7.

48. Trojani C, Beaufils P, Burdin G, et al. Revision ACL reconstruction: influence of a lateral tenodesis. Knee Surg Sports Traumatol Arthrosc 2012;20:1565–70.

49. Ferretti A, Conteduca F, Monaco E, et al. Revision anterior cruciate ligament reconstruction with doubled semitendinosus and gracilis tendons and lateral extra-articular reconstruction. Surgical technique. J Bone Joint Surg Am 2007; 89(Suppl 2 Pt.2):196–213.

50. Musahl V, Kopf S, Rabuck S, et al. Rotatory knee laxity tests and the pivot shift as tools for ACL treatment algorithm. Knee Surg Sports Traumatol Arthrosc 2012;20:793–800.

51. Vundelinckx B, Herman B, Getgood A, et al. Surgical indications and technique for anterior cruciate ligament reconstruction combined with lateral extra-articular tenodesis or anterolateral ligament reconstruction. Clin Sports Med 2017;36(1):135–53.

52. Wascher DC, Lording TD, Neyret P. Extra-articular procedures for the ACL-deficient knee: a state of the art review. JISAKOS 2016;1–9.

53. Lording TD, Lustig S, Servien E, et al. Lateral reinforcement in anterior cruciate-ligament reconstruction. Sports Med Arthrosc Rehabil Ther Technol 2014;1:3–10.

54. Lemaire M. Ruptures an ciennes du ligament croise anterieur du genou. J Chir 1967;93:311–20.

55. Christel P, Djian P. Anterio-lateral extra-articular tenodesis of the knee using a short strip of fascia lata. Rev Chir Orthop Reparatrice Appar Mot 2002;88:508–13.

56. Ellison AE. Distal iliotibial-band transfer for anterolateral rotatory instability of the knee. J Bone Joint Surg Am 1979;61:330–7.

57. Macintosh D, Darby T. Lateral substitution reconstruction. In: Proceedings of the Canadian Orthopaedic Association. J Bone Joint Surg Br 1976;58(1):142.

58. Arnold JA, Coker TP, Heaton LM, et al. Natural history of anterior cruciate tears. Am J Sports Med 1979;7:305–13.

59. Losee RE, Johnson TR, Southwick WO. Anterior subluxation of the lateral tibial plateau. A diagnostic test and operative repair. J Bone Joint Surg Am 1978;60:1015–30.

60. Andrews JR, Sanders RA. "Mini-reconstruction" technique in treating anterolateral rotatory instability (ALRI). Clin Orthop Relat Res 1983;172:93–6.
61. Kennedy JC, Stewart R, Walker DM. Anterolateral rotatory instability of the knee joint. J Bone Joint Surg Am 1978;60:1031–9.
62. Fox JM, Blazina ME, Del Pizzo W, et al. Extra-articular stabilization of the knee joint for anterior instability. Clin Orthop Relat Res 1980;147:56–61.
63. Ireland J, Trickey E. MacIntosh tenodesis for anterolateral instability of the knee. J Bone Jt Surg Br 1980;62:340–5.
64. Amirault JD, Cameron JC, MacIntosh DL, et al. Chronic anterior cruciate ligament deficiency. Long-term results of MacIntosh's lateral substitution reconstruction. J Bone Joint Surg Br 1988;70(4):622–4.
65. Sydney S, Haynes D, Hungerford D, et al. The altered kinematic effect of an ilitotibial band tenodesis on the anterior cruciate deficient knee. Trans Orthopd Res Soc Annu Meet 1987;340.
66. Draganich LF, Reider B, Miller PR. An in vitro study of the Muller anterolateral femorotibial ligament tenodesis in the anterior cruciate ligament deficient knee. Am J Sports Med 1989;17:357–62.
67. Strum GM, Fox JM, Ferkel RD, et al. Intraarticular versus intraarticular and extra-articular reconstruction for chronic anterior cruciate ligament instability. Clin Orthop Relat Res 1989;245:188–98.
68. Marcacci M, Zaffagnini S, Iacono F, et al. Arthroscopic intra- and extra-articular anterior cruciate ligament reconstruction with gracilis and semitendinosus tendons. Knee Surg Sports Traumatol Arthrosc 1998;6:68–75.
69. Colombet PD. Navigated intra-articular ACL reconstruction with additional extra-articular tenodesis using the same hamstring graft. Knee Surg Sports Traumatol Arthrosc 2011;19:384–9.
70. Marshall JL, Warren RF, Wickiewicz TL, et al. The anterior cruciate ligament: a technique of repair and reconstruction. Clin Orthop Relat Res 1979;143:97–106.
71. Lerat JL, Duprã La Tour L, Herzberg G, et al. Review of 100 patients operated on for chronic anterior laxity of the knee by a procedure derived from the Jones and MacIntosh methods. Value of dynamic radiography for the objective analysis of the results. Rev Chir Orthop Reparatrice Appar Mot 1987;73(Suppl 2):201–4.
72. Zarins B, Rowe CR. Combined anterior cruciate-ligament reconstruction using semitendinosus tendon and iliotibial tract. J Bone Joint Surg Am 1986;68:160–77.
73. O'Brien SJ, Warren RF, Wickiewicz TL, et al. The iliotibial band lateral sling procedure and its effect on the results of anterior cruciate ligament reconstruction. Am J Sports Med 1991;19:21–4.
74. Marcacci M, Zaffagnini S, Giordano G, et al. Anterior cruciate ligament reconstruction associated with extra-articular tenodesis: a prospective clinical and radiographic evaluation with 10- to 13-year follow-up. Am J Sports Med 2009;37:707–14.
75. Pernin J, Verdonk P, Si Selmi TA, et al. Long-term follow-up of 24.5 years after intra-articular anterior cruciate ligament reconstruction with lateral extra-articular augmentation. Am J Sports Med 2010;38:1094–102.
76. Saragaglia D, Pison A, Refaie R. Lateral tenodesis combined with anterior cruciate ligament reconstruction using a unique semitendinosus and gracilis transplant. Int Orthop 2013;37(8):1575–81.
77. Ferretti A, Monaco E, Ponzo A, et al. Combined intra-articular and extra-articular reconstruction in anterior cruciate ligament-deficient knee: 25 years later. Arthroscopy 2016;32(10):2039–47.

78. Guzzini M, Mazza D, Fabbri M, et al. Extra-articular tenodesis combined with an anterior cruciate ligament reconstruction in acute anterior cruciate ligament tear in elite female football players. Int Orthop 2016;40(10):2091–6.

79. Dodds AL, Gupte CM, Neyret P, et al. Extra-articular techniques in anterior cruciate ligament reconstruction: a literature review. J Bone Joint Surg Br 2011;93: 1440–8.

80. Rezende FC, De Moraes VY, Martimbianco AL, et al. Does combined intra- and extraarticular ACL reconstruction improve function and stability? A meta-analysis. Clin Orthop Relat Res 2015;473:2609–18.

81. Song GY, Hong L, Zhang H, et al. Clinical outcomes of combined lateral extra-articular tenodesis and intra-articular anterior cruciate ligament reconstruction in addressing high-grade pivot-shift phenomenon. Arthroscopy 2016;32(5): 898–905.

82. Smith JO, Yasen SK, Lord B, et al. Combined anterolateral ligament and anatomic anterior cruciate ligament reconstruction of the knee. Knee Surg Sports Traumatol Arthrosc 2015;23:3151–6.

83. Helito CP, Bonadio MB, Gobbi RG, et al. Combined intra- and extra-articular reconstruction of the anterior cruciate ligament: the reconstruction of the knee anterolateral ligament. Arthrosc Tech 2015;4:239–44.

84. Helito CP, Demange MK, Bonadio MB, et al. Radiographic landmarks for locating the femoral origin and tibial insertion of the knee anterolateral ligament. Am J Sports Med 2014;42:2356–62.

85. Sonnery-Cottet B, Daggett M, Helito CP, et al. Combined anterior cruciate ligament and anterolateral ligament reconstruction. Arthrosc Tech 2016;5(6): e1253–9.

86. Wagih AM, Elguindy AM. Percutaneous reconstruction of the anterolateral ligament of the knee with a polyester tape. Arthrosc Tech 2016;5(4):691–7.

87. Sonnery-Cottet B, Saithna A, Cavalier M, et al. Anterolateral ligament reconstruction is associated with significantly reduced ACL graft rupture rates at a minimum follow-up of 2 years. Am J Sports Med 2017;45(7):1547–57.

88. Zhang H, Qiu M, Zhou A, et al. Anatomic anterolateral ligament reconstruction improves postoperative clinical outcomes combined with anatomic anterior cruciate ligament reconstruction. J Sports Sci Med 2016;15(4):688–96.

The Role of an Extra-Articular Tenodesis in Revision of Anterior Cruciate Ligament Reconstruction

Thomas K. Miller, MD

KEYWORDS

- High-grade laxity • Pivot shift • Iliotibial tract • Anterolateral ligament • ACL revision
- Extra-articular tenodesis

KEY POINTS

- Despite modern techniques and a technically well-positioned anterior cruciate ligament (ACL) graft, failure can still occur.
- Patients with high-grade ligamentous laxity are at increased risk for ACL graft failure.
- Iliotibial tract tenodesis should be considered as an ACL revision adjunct in select patients.
- Anterolateral ligament reconstruction or lateral extra-articular tenodesis is contraindicated in patients with posterolateral corner injuries or lateral compartment degenerative joint disease.

INTRODUCTION

Although an intraarticular anterior cruciate ligament (ACL) reconstruction using current methods can be expected to result in a reliable knee and allow return to activities as desired,[1–3] some patients will experience graft failure[4,5] and require revision surgery.[6–10] Although most failures are secondary to technical errors, a subset of patients will have residual objective or subjective instability expressed by a persistent pivot shift or lateral rotatory instability despite a well-positioned graft of appropriate size and managed with an acceptable postoperative rehabilitation program.[11,12] When assessing revision options for this group of reconstruction failures,[13–16] those patients with generalized joint laxity[17,18] and revisions requiring the use of soft tissue grafts, the addition of a lateral extra-articular tenodesis should be considered as a possible adjunct to the intraarticular revision component of the procedure.[19–23] A lateral stabilization procedure should not be used to supplement the intraarticular component of

Department of Orthopaedic Surgery, Virginia Tech/Carilion School of Medicine, Institute for Orthopaedics and Neurosciences, 2331 Franklin Road, Roanoke, VA 24018, USA
E-mail address: tkmiller@carilionclinic.org

Clin Sports Med 37 (2018) 101–113
http://dx.doi.org/10.1016/j.csm.2017.07.010
0278-5919/18/© 2017 Elsevier Inc. All rights reserved.

the revision in patients with posterolateral corner injuries[15] and lateral compartment articular compromise.[24–26] Regardless of the extra-articular procedure selected, just as with the intraarticular revision, the impact of prior surgical approaches, skin quality, retained hardware, bone loss, and the intraarticular revision itself may impact the feasibility and value of the extra-articular supplement.[2,27–31] The addition of an extra-articular procedure, although not a "cure all" for ACL revision challenges, may be the adjunctive reconstruction component necessary to provide sufficient improvement in rotational stability that leads to an improved functional outcome for a select subset of patients.

In the United States, it is estimated that approximately 175,000 to 330,000 ACL injuries occur per year with 75 to 100,000 ACL reconstructions performed annually.[1,32] Acceptable outcomes for ACL reconstructions using current surgical techniques are reported in between 75% and 90%[1–3] of primary ACL procedures.

Although intraarticular reconstructions are associated with generally acceptable outcomes,[1–3,33] as reflected by improvement in laxity and return to activities, International Knee Documentation Committee scores after reconstruction are generally between 80% and 95%[1] with persistent instability reported in 11% to 30% of patients and dissatisfaction after reconstruction is often associated with a residual positive pivot shift or complaints of abnormal mechanics during activities.[34–38] Biau and colleagues[39] reported that 32% of autograft ACL reconstructions had a persistent positive Lachman test and 22% had a positive Pivot after reconstruction. The MOON group has reported a 4.4% failure rate at 2 years and progression to 7.7% at 6 years.[4,5] Failure to restore joint kinematics is higher than generally expected and the actual incidence of reconstruction failure, for a variety of reasons, is most likely underreported.[40]

Tibor's review of trends in ACL techniques from 2007 to 2014 quotes a consistent rate of revision at 2.3%, despite the evolution in preferred operative techniques[8,9] during this time frame.[41] The rate of ACL reconstruction revision is reported to range from 3.1% according to the Swedish National Registry Study of 17,000 plus reconstructions[6] to 4.1% rate of revision according to the Danish registry[10] and as high as 8.4% as reported by Yabroudi and colleagues.[7] These estimated rates of revision range from as few as 3000 to as many as 10,000 ACL revision procedures per year.[42,43]

As described by several authors, failure can be defined in a number of manners, including pain, stiffness, extensor mechanism dysfunction, infection,[44,45] inability to return to sports,[46] and, for the purposes of this discussion, objective laxity or patient perception of residual instability when performing sports or daily activities.[2] Although residual laxity or instability is most commonly associated with graft failure owing to technical causes[47] (and reported in as many as 77%-95% of failures seen within 6 months of surgery),[32] unrecognized or untreated associated instability increases the load on the ACL graft during the early healing and revascularization phase with the potential for graft compromise.[2] Untreated ligamentous laxity has been reported to occur in 7%[47] to 15% of ACL graft failures.[48] The most common associated ligamentous injury is medial collateral ligament injury seen in 20% of knees with an ACL injury[49] and posterolateral corner injuries are reported in up to 15% of chronic ACL-deficient knees.[50] However, the presence of residual lateral rotational instability, as defined by the presence of a persistent pivot shift, has been the instability pattern often linked to patient dissatisfaction and associated compromises in ability to return to sports.[51]

A well-performed ACL reconstruction, using current techniques of graft placement and appropriate graft selection, can be expected to lead to control of the pivot shift[1] in the presence of intact lateral structures.[13] It is, however, recognized that, despite the generally good outcomes with an isolated intraarticular graft, failures are seen without what might be considered obvious errors in technique, subsequent postoperative management,[11] or timing of return to activities. The impact of this subtle and perhaps undertreated laxity on ACL instability has led to renewed interest in the historically reported contribution of the iliotibial tract (or anterolateral ligament) to stability[52–56] and the role of lateral tenodesis in the management of ACL instability.[27,57–63]

As stated by Galway and MacIntosh, the "sine qua non of the lateral pivot shift is a torn ACL."[64] Noted in the same publication was the variable impact on the pattern of instability and pivot shift owing to concomitant iliotibial tract injury. Acute anterolateral instability of the knee was described by Norwood in 1979[53] followed by a comprehensive classification of lateral injuries and associated instability patterns by Hughston and coworkers.[54] The presence of iliotibial tract injuries in association with an ACL disruption and the impact of such injuries was reported by Terry and associates[52] in 1993. These investigators reported findings of a 93% occurrence has been confirmed by subsequent studies by Ferretti and colleagues, who found such injuries in 90% of "isolated" ACL injured knees.[33] MRI studies have shown that iliotibial tract and anterolateral ligament damage can be visualized in 32%[52] or more of knees with ACL injuries.[57]

According to Terry and colleagues, the spectrum of injury to the iliotibial tract would account for variations in the clinical examination of the ACL-injured knee.[52] The role of the lateral extra-articular restraints (based on sectioning studies) was summarized by Wroble and associates[65] and the contribution of the iliotibial tract and anterolateral ligament injury to the severity of pivot shift, particularly in grade II and grade III instability by Tanaka and colleagues, and other investigators.[66–68] Such lateral tract deficiency and subsequent instability is felt to be result from the primary injury or may occur owing to attenuation from chronic repetitive episodes ofinstability.[69]Recent work by Noyes and associates[70] confirmed that an isolated ACL tear could result in a pivot shift. However, when combined with a complete loss of the anterolateral ligament and iliotibial band was associated with a severe or grade 3 pivot shift. Echoing Terry and associates[52] and other investigators[42] was the opinion that there was "considerable variation in rotational stability between knees with the same anatomic injury."[70]

The work by Trojani and coworkers,[22] which showed a reduction in the occurrence of pivot in augmented versus nonaugmented ACL reconstructions, seems to support the value of lateral tenodesis, especially in those with significant lateral tract deficiency.[71] However, the magnitude of the contribution of the lateral structures to the control of tibial rotation is limited and, per Thein and colleagues, only when the tibia has displaced beyond that seen in an intact ACL.[72] Or to summarize, although the pivot shift requires a torn ACL,[64,70] a torn ACL does not necessarily imply that a pivot shift will be present on examination[65,73] and the contribution of an iliotibial tract injury and/or anterolateral ligament injury may account for this variability[70] and the severity of the pivot shift.

Even if an anterolateral ligament injury occurs, there is a strong sentiment, as summarized by Noyes and coworkers, that a well-performed ACL reconstruction is sufficient to provide appropriate knee stability in the majority of patients.[24] This conclusion is supported the metaanalysis performed by Rezende and coworkers,[20] which showed no difference when comparing isolated ACL reconstructions to a reconstructions with extra-articular augmentation in International Knee Documentation Committee score, return to activity and Tegner Lysholm scores. Opposing sentiment has been published by several others reporting that a residual symptomatic pivot shift may be seen in 10% to 30% of patients after isolated intraarticular procedure ACL reconstructions.[35,36,74]

Several factors, when taken together, support the consideration of a lateral supplement when planning revision ACL procedures. The report by Magnussen[75] showed that the presence of high-grade laxity as defined by high-grade pivot shift, anterior drawer or Lachman test, increased the odds reconstruction failure and the need for subsequent revision ACL reconstruction surgery. Persistence of abnormal tibial rotation is seen in some patients after isolated intraarticular ACL reconstruction.[35] A reduction of pivot shift can be seen when an extra-articular tenodesis is performed in conjunction with an intraarticular ACL reconstruction.[22] Subsequently, when assessing options in revision ACL surgery, the addition of a lateral tenodesis or reconstruction procedure merits consideration[14,16] and should be a component of the reconstruction armamentarium for a select subset of patients.[13,15]

In general, a revision ACL reconstruction must be viewed as a salvage procedure.[76] Although acceptable objective results are possible,[73,77] outcomes based on both objective and subjective criteria regarding stability or return to desired activities is less favorable than after primary ACL reconstruction[10,43,77,78] with a success rate of 87%[79] in revision surgery as compared with 92% in primary surgery.[32] The metaanalysis by Wright and colleagues[80] determined that revision ACL reconstruction is associated with poor results when compared with primary ACL reconstruction with both lower patient reported outcomes and an objective failure rate of 13.75%, which is significantly higher than that of primary ACL reconstruction.

Accurate identification of the cause of failure is essential to determining the best revision strategy[32] and, given the challenges in obtaining acceptable results in revision surgery, small modifications or additions to the reconstructive "package" may make a substantial difference in outcomes.

With that consideration, the question becomes, "is there role for and what patient subset may benefit from the addition of a lateral tenodesis as a component of a revision ACL reconstruction." Once all the other "usual" factors leading to reconstruction failure have been considered, a rationale for the inclusion of a lateral tenodesis procedure in revision ACL reconstruction was well stated by McGuire as being an appropriate consideration for patients with a failed isolated ACL reconstruction in which "the tunnels, the graft, and the rehabilitation have all been done properly."[12] This concept has also been extended to the rerevision subgroup.[81,82]

Determination of the most appropriate reconstruction plan, although dictated by recognition and attention to the commonly referenced modifiable causes of recurrent instability, must begin, as with the planning of any ACL reconstruction, with a determination of the severity and pattern of instability. Although a well-placed intraarticular graft can be expected to restore stability in the majority of patients and numerous studies have reported that there is no residual internal rotation abnormality when anterolateral structures are intact,[19,71,83] when anterolateral deficiency is present, residual abnormality in the lateral translation can persist.[19,71] Given the potential contribution of lateral compromise to instability as reflected by a severe pivot shift[66,67] and the potential contribution of this instability to subsequent reconstruction failure,[35,75,84] preoperative planning for revision surgery must include (when possible) a determination of the initial examination with regard to the Lachman test, pivot shift, and drawer severity. Those patients with a severe pivot shift before the index reconstruction may have objective or subjective residual after reconstruction instability owing to a failure to address the secondary instability pattern (owing to lateral structure injury) even with a well-performed, isolated intraarticular graft procedure.[35,85,86] Because a reduction in pivot shift has been documented with the addition of a lateral extra-articular tenodesis,[20,87] if the index examination indicated severe instability (left untreated) or the current examination indicates severe instability, adjunctive measures such as lateral tenodesis should be considered as an adjunctive procedure in the revision planning.[14,22] The use of a lateral reconstruction as a supplement to the intraarticular graft in revision surgery has been shown to reduce both Lachman test and pivot shift[22,23] as compared with an isolated intraarticular graft procedure with improvement in both Lysholm and Tegner scores[23] and is independent of the graft used.[22] In light of the generally poor outcomes and failures rates in revision surgery, Trojani and associates[22] also felt that the lateral tenodesis showed a tendency toward reduced revision failure compared with nonsupplemented revision techniques. To summarize, the primary indication for the addition of an extra-articular tenodesis is in patients with severe initial or postreconstruction instability as shown by a grade 3 or higher Lachman test, and especially grade 3 pivot shift. This subset of reconstruction failures should be considered candidates for the inclusion of an extra-articular tenodesis as an adjunct to the intraarticular graft procedure.

Similarly, those with generalized joint laxity may be considered as an at "at-risk" group if requiring revision surgery. As reported by Akhtar and colleagues,[17] patients with generalized joint laxity had a higher risk of requiring revision surgery, often without clear reason for graft failure. Studies by Kim and associates[18] indicate that hamstring autografts and even bone–tendon–bone autografts may be insufficient to manage instability in this group of patients. When a primary reconstruction has been unsuccessful, with or without gross lateral insufficiency[16] on index or postfailure examination, this group of patients would also seem to be candidates for inclusion of a lateral tenodesis as a "belt and suspenders" approach to reduce the severity of overall laxity and reduce lateral translation to offload the intraarticular revision component.

The graft used for the index reconstruction and the impact of graft availability and selection for a revision procedure may also lead to consideration of lateral supplementation. A metaanalysis by Biau and coworkers[88] showed that autograft patellar tendon graft had a significantly decreased risk of a positive pivot shift when compared with hamstring in primary ACL reconstruction. Per Rezende and associates,[20] the addition of an extra-articular procedure did not show superior stability when bone–tendon–bone was the graft used (as compared with autograft hamstring) in a primary reconstruction. Unfortunately, a bone–tendon–bone autograft may not be available or appropriate for use in many revision procedures. The ipsilateral bone–tendon–bone autograft may have already been used for the index reconstruction and contralateral bone–tendon–bone may not be an option for a variety of reasons (contralateral reconstruction, insufficient size of graft, bone loss mandating larger graft bone stock, patient preference). Modifications to the operative approach may be required to avoid prior tunnels or retained hardware, bone loss, and compromises in fixation options may also impact graft options. As a result, the use of soft tissue grafts—autograft hamstring or allograft (soft tissue, bone–tendon–bone, or Achilles)—may become the default choice to accommodate any of these issues. Balanced against the need to select a soft tissue graft choice are concerns of graft failure in the use of isolated hamstring autografts owing to potential failure secondary to graft creep[89] and potentially less reliable and longer incorporation time compared with bone–tendon–bone for soft tissue autografts.[90,91] Because failure to restore abnormalities in tibial rotation has been reported with the use of autograft hamstring grafts,[86] lateral supplementation has been proposed for this graft group in revision surgery.[20,92] Similarly, allograft material also been associated with concerns about graft failure owing to longer incorporation time as compared with bone–tendon–bone,[93] and has been associated with a higher incidence of recurrent instability when compared with autograft materials.[84]

The addition of an extra-articular tenodesis (and resultant limitation of lateral rotation) has been proposed as a means of offloading and protecting soft tissue grafts during healing and revascularization[92] owing to a reduction of graft load by as much as 43%,[19] and is considered to be of value to protect the allograft tissue in anterior cruciate reconstruction including revision procedures.[21] Although the number of patients reviewed has been small, revision surgery using a hamstring autograft when performed in combination with a lateral procedure, has been reported to restore stability[23] and shows improvement in pivot shift.[22] Because the addition of an extra-articular procedure has been reported to add superior stability for anterior cruciate ligament reconstructions performed with hamstring autografts[20] and, given the concerns associated with these graft options and the potential impact of residual instability on graft healing, if soft tissue grafts are required for the revision procedure, adjunctive lateral surgery to "protect" the graft during incorporation and revascularization is an appropriate consideration.

Despite the best preoperative planning for revision procedures, compromises are inevitable.

The use of staged procedures to address hardware interference, bone deficit or tunnel overlap, optimal graft selection, and flexibility in the surgical approach may still not allow ideal graft placement within the ACL footprint.[21] Although it has been reported that transtibial or nonanatomic graft placement can lead to acceptable results[6,61] and even over the top or other nonanatomic procedures may need to be considered,[94,95] the addition of the lateral tenodesis to control rotation and reduce pivot shift in cases of unavoidable suboptimal graft position may be of benefit[15] to "salvage" a revision procedure by offloading the graft[19] and improving subjective sensation of stability.

An extremely small subset of patients may exist where an intraarticular reconstruction has controlled anterior translation, the graft is intact and yet rotational instability persists.[35] Anterior translation may be acceptable but rotational instability, objective and subjective, impacts knee function and reliability. If the graft can be confirmed as intact and sufficient to control sagittal stability (direct examination with less than 4–5 mm side to side difference, with MRI and/or arthroscopic assessment confirmation of an intact graft) and the patient complaints are of the rotational instability, a lateral supplement may be of value and may be sufficient to control the subtle yet clinically problematic rotational insufficiency[15] without an intraarticular revision.

The addition of a lateral procedure cannot be viewed as a panacea, and there is subset of patients with failed anterior cruciate reconstructions for whom addition of a lateral procedure is contraindicated.

As noted, untreated concomitant instability as a cause of reconstruction failure[47,48] must be recognized. Although the use of a lateral tenodesis merits consideration as a means to address such instability in a select subset of such patients (those with lateral rotatory instability), it must be recognized that the presence of posterolateral laxity is seen in as high of 15% of ACL injuries and is the most common untreated coexisting laxity associated with residual dysfunction after ACL reconstruction.[50] The (abnormal) tibial position associated with posterolateral corner injury is reflected in the external rotation recurvatum test with an increased external rotation tibial position and recurvatum. Anterolateral ligament or iliotibial band reconstructive procedures require fixation in a position of lateral and external tibial rotation with compromise of the normal screw home mechanism.[19] The addition of a reconstruction requiring external tibial rotation during graft tensioning and fixation, as required for an anterolateral ligament reconstruction and iliotibial tract tenodesis, would serve to compound the posterolateral corner injury associated malposition by constraining the tibia in a subluxated position and is, therefore, contraindicated when posterolateral corner insufficiency is present.[15]

Despite the recommendation by Andrews and colleagues[27] that a lateral tenodesis should address excessive rotation but not compromise range of motion, the addition of a lateral tenodesis using current techniques generally does constraint tibial rotation,[19,36] and has the potential to increase joint load.[3] Concerns have been expressed that such overconstraint[3,96] will increase the risk of degenerative joint changes and progression of joint arthrosis has been reported in combined intraarticular and extra-articular procedures.[25,26] For those patients with a significant pivot shift as a component of their instability pattern but with documented lateral compartment degenerative disease or after lateral meniscectomy, the addition of a lateral tenodesis must carefully weigh the balance of reduction of lateral translation with the potential acceleration of degenerative joint disease.

Just as there has been an evolution of surgical procedures to address anterior cruciate injuries, the rationale for and "optimal" procedure to address iliotibial tract insufficiency is not well-defined. Historical procedures,[27,58,59] modifications,[23] or other procedures[21] are considerations in the addition of a lateral tenodesis procedure as a revision adjunct. Regardless of debate associated with the preferred or optimal extra-articular procedure, factors associated with the revision "package" may impact the potential for its inclusion in a revision scenario. Prior operative approaches and skin quality must be taken in to account and the impact of prior surgical approaches may add unacceptable morbidity[29] to the addition of a lateral procedure. Even the use of so called mini approaches[27,28] to avoid skin compromise may not permit addition of a lateral tenodesis. As with the intra articular component of a revision, "real estate and hardware" issues may come in to play.[2] Bone deficiency,[30] the impact of hardware not removed,[31] and the potential for condyle fracture may require consideration of suboptimal position or fixation of the tenodesis or may result in the complete inability to add the lateral supplement.

SUMMARY

Although most ACL reconstruction failures are due to readily identifiable errors in technique, some apparently well-positioned and appropriately sized grafts fail with objective signs or patient complaints of instability. For patients with a severe pivot shift, an intraarticular ACL procedure may not be sufficient to control the associated instability, and may impact graft healing and lead to graft failure and instability. Patients with a high-grade pivot shift at the time of the index procedure and subsequent reconstruction failure or a high-grade pivot shift present at the time of revision surgery as well as patients with generalized joint laxity and reconstruction failure should be considered candidates for the inclusion of a lateral tenodesis procedure to supplement the intraarticular revision graft. Revisions requiring soft tissue grafts or suboptimal graft placement owing to the inherent issues associated with revision procedures may also benefit from lateral tenodesis to offload the intraarticular graft during healing. Owing to the tibial positioning associated with tensioning and fixation of extra-articular procedures, the addition a lateral tenodesis should not be used in patients with posterolateral corner injuries, lateral meniscus loss, or lateral compartment articular disease.

The addition of an extra-articular tenodesis cannot be viewed as a "cure all" and does not replace appropriate planning and attention to all aspects relating to a reconstruction failure and the complex requirements associated with a successful revision procedure. In a select subset of patients, however, the addition of an extra-articular tenodesis to address rotational instability may lead to an improved functional outcome in ACL revision surgery.

REFERENCES

1. Hofbauer M, Muller B, Murawski CD, et al. The concept of individualized anatomic ligament (ACL) reconstruction. Knee Surg Sports Traumatol Arthrosc 2014;22:979–86.
2. Kamath GV, Redfern JC, Greis PE, et al. Revision anterior ligament reconstruction. Am J Sports Med 2011;39:199–217.
3. Slette EL, Mikula JD, Schon JM, et al. Biomechanical results of lateral extra-articular tenodesis procedures of the knee: a systematic review. Arthroscopy 2016;32:2592–611.
4. Hettrich CM, Dunn WR, Reinke EK, et al. The rate of subsequent surgery and predictors after anterior cruciate ligament reconstruction: two and 6 year follow-up from a multicenter cohort. Am J Sports Med 2013;41:1534–40.
5. Kaeding CC, Pedroza AD, Reinke EK, et al. MOON consortium. Risk factors and predictors of subsequent ACL injury in either knee after ACL reconstruction: prospective analysis of 2488 primary ACL reconstructions from the MOON cohort. Am J Sports Med 2015;43:1583–90.
6. Desai N, Andernord D, Sundemo D, et al. Revision surgery in anterior cruciate ligament reconstruction: a cohort study of 17,682 patients from the Swedish national knee ligament register. Knee Surg Sports Traumatol Arthrosc 2017;25(5): 1542–54.
7. Yabroudi MA, Bjornsson H, Lynch AD, et al. Predictors of revision surgery after primary anterior cruciate ligament reconstruction. Orthop J Sports Med 2016;4: 1–7.
8. Garrett WE Jr, Swiontkowski MF, Weinstein JN, et al. American Board of Orthopaedic Surgery practice of the orthopaedic surgeon: part -II, certification exam mix. J Bone Joint Surg Am 2006;88:660–7.
9. Leathers MP, Merz A, Wong J, et al. Trends and demographics in anterior cruciate ligament reconstruction in the United States. J Knee Surg 2015;28:390–4.
10. Lind M, Menhart F, Pederson AB. Incidence and outcome after revision anterior cruciate ligament reconstruction: results from the Danish registry for knee ligament reconstructions. Am J Sports Med 2012;40:1551–7.
11. Frank RM, McGill KC, Cole BJ, et al. An institution-specific analysis of ACL reconstruction failure. J Knee Surg 2012;25:143–9.
12. McGuire DA, Wolchok J. Extra-articular lateral reconstruction technique. Arthroscopy 2000;16:553–7.
13. Butler PD, Mellecker CJ, Rudert MJ, et al. Single-bundle versus double-bundle ALC reconstructions in isolation and in conjunction with extra-articular iliotibial band tenodesis. Iowa Orthop J 2013;33:97–104.
14. Colosimo AJ, Heidt RS, Traub JA, et al. Revision anterior cruciate ligament surgery with a reharvested ipsilateral patellar tendon. Am J Sports Med 2001;29: 746–50.
15. Magnussen RA, Lustig S, Matthias M, et al. The role of extra-articular reconstruction in revision ACL reconstruction. In: Marx RG, editor. Revision ACL reconstruction: indications and technique. New York: Springer; 2014. p. 151–6.
16. Dodds AL, Gupte CM, Neyret P, et al. Extra-articular techniques in anterior cruciate ligament reconstruction, a literature review. J Bone Joint Surg Br 2011;93: 1440–8.
17. Akhtar MA, Bhattacharya R, Keating JF. Generalized ligamentous laxity and revision ACL surgery: is there a relation? Knee 2016;23(6):1148–53.

18. Kim SJ, Kumar P, Kim SH. Anterior cruciate ligament reconstruction in patients with generalized joint laxity. Clin Orthop Surg 2010;2:130–9.
19. Engebretsen L, Lew WD, Lewis JL, et al. The effect of an iliotibial tenodesis on intraarticular graft forces and knee motion. Am J Sports Med 1990;18:169–76.
20. Rezende FC, de Moraes VY, Martimbianco AL, et al. Does combined intra- and extraarticular ACL reconstruction improve function and stability? A meta-analysis. Clin Orthop Relat Res 2015;473:2609–18.
21. Mascarenhas R, McConkey MO, Forsythe B, et al. Revision anterior cruciate ligament reconstruction with bone-patellar tendon-bone allograft and extra-articular iliotibial band tenodesis. Am J Orthop (Belle Mead NJ) 2015;44:E89–92.
22. Trojani C, Beaufils P, Burdin G, et al. Revision ACL reconstruction: influence of a lateral tenodesis. Knee Surg Sports Traumatol Arthrosc 2012;21:690–5.
23. Ferretti A, Conteduca F, Monaco E, et al. Revision anterior cruciate ligament reconstruction with doubled semitendinosus and gracilis tendons and lateral extra-articular reconstruction. J Bone Joint Surg Am 2006;88:2373–9.
24. Noyes FR. Editorial commentary: lateral extra-articular reconstruction with anterior cruciate ligament surgery: are these operative procedures supported by in vitro biomechanical studies? Arthroscopy 2016;32:2612–5.
25. Roth JH, Kennedy JC, Lockstadt H, et al. Intra articular reconstruction of the anterior cruciate ligament with and without extra-articular supplementation by transfer of the biceps tendon. J Bone Joint Surg Am 1987;69:275–8.
26. Strum GM, Fox JM, Ferkel RD, et al. Intraarticular versus intraarticular and extra-articular reconstruction for chronic anterior cruciate ligament instability. Clin Orthop Relat Res 1989;(245):188–98.
27. Andrews JR, Sanders RA, Morin B. Surgical treatment of anterolateral rotatory instability. Am J Sports Med 1985;13:112–9.
28. Khiami F, Wajsfisz A, Meyer A, et al. Anterior cruciate ligament reconstruction with fascia lata using a minimally invasive arthroscopic harvesting technique. Orthop Traumatol Surg Res 2013;99:99–105.
29. Wetzler MJ, Bartolozzi AR, Gillespie MJ. Revision anterior cruciate ligament reconstruction. Oper Tech Sports Med 1996;6:181–91.
30. Maak TG, Voos JE, Wickiewicz TL, et al. Tunnel widening in revision anterior cruciate ligament reconstruction. J Am Acad Orthop Surg 2010;18:695–706.
31. Maak TG, Delos D, Cordasco FA. Preoperative planning for revision ACL reconstruction. In: Marx RG, editor. Revision ACL reconstruction: indications and technique. New York: Springer; 2014. p. 63–74.
32. Di Benedetto P, Di Benedetto E, Fiocchi A, et al. Causes of failure of anterior cruciate ligament reconstruction and revision surgical strategies. Knee Surg Relat Res 2016;28:319–24.
33. Ferretti A, Monaco E, Fabbri M, et al. Prevalence and classification of injuries of the anterolateral complex in acute anterior cruciate ligament tears. Arthroscopy 2017;33:147–54.
34. Monaco E, Maestri B, Conteduca F, et al. Extra-articular reconstruction and pivot shift: in vivo dynamic evaluation with navigation. Am J Sports Med 2014;42:1669–74.
35. Tashman S, Collon D, Anderson K, et al. Abnormal rotational motion during running after anterior cruciate ligament reconstruction. Am J Sports Med 2004;32:975–83.
36. Anderson AF, Snyder RB, Libscomb AB Jr. Anterior cruciate ligament reconstruction. A prospective randomized study of three surgical methods. Am J Sports Med 2001;29:272–9.

37. Aglietti P, Buzzi R, Giron F, et al. Arthroscopic-assisted anterior cruciate ligament reconstruction with central third patellar tendon. A 5-8 year follow-up. Knee Surg Sports Traumatol Arthrosc 1997;5:138–44.
38. Bach BR Jr, Tradonsky S, Bojchuk J, et al. Arthroscopically assisted anterior cruciate ligament reconstruction using patellar tendon autograft. Five to Nine – year follow up evaluation. Am J Sports Med 1998;8:1–6.
39. Biau DJ, Tournoux C, Katsahian S, et al. Bone-patellar tendon- bone autografts versus hamstring autografts for reconstruction of the anterior cruciate ligament: meta-analysis. BMJ 2006;332:995–1001.
40. Gianotti SM, Marshall SW, Hume PA, et al. Incidence of anterior cruciate ligament injury and other knee ligament injuries: a national population-based study. J Sci Med Sport 2009;12:622–7.
41. Tibor L, Chan P, Funahashi TT, et al. Surgical technique trend in primary ACL reconstruction from 2007 to 2014. J Bone Joint Surg Am 2016;98:1079–89.
42. Fox JA, Pierce M, Bojchuk J, et al. Revision anterior cruciate ligament reconstruction with nonirradiated fresh- frozen patellar tendon allograft. Arthroscopy 2004; 20:787–94.
43. Noyes FR, Barber-Westin SDS. Revision anterior cruciate ligament reconstruction: report of 11-year experience and results in 114 patients. Instr Course Lect 2001;50:451–61.
44. Van Eck CF, Schreiber VM, Liu TT, et al. The anatomic approach to primary, revision and augmentation anterior cruciate ligament reconstruction. Knee Surg Sports Traumatol Arthrosc 2010;17:1154–63.
45. Johnson DL, Coen MJ. Revision ACL surgery. Etiology, Indications, techniques and results. Am J Knee Surg 1995;8:145–67.
46. Adern CL, Webster KE, Taylor NF, et al. Return to sport following anterior cruciate ligament reconstruction: a systematic review and meta-analysis of the state of play. Br J Sports Med 2011;45:596–606.
47. MARS Group, Wright RW, Huston LJ, Spindler KP, et al. Descriptive epidemiology of the multicenter ACL revision study (MARS) cohort. Am J Sports Med 2010;38: 1979–86.
48. Getelman MH, Friedman MJ. Revision anterior cruciate ligament reconstruction surgery. J Am Acad Orthop Surg 1999;7:189–98.
49. Yoon KH, Yoo JH, Kim KI. Bone contusion and associated meniscal and medial collateral ligament injury in patient with anterior cruciate ligament rupture. J Bone Joint Surg Am 2001;93:1510–8.
50. LaPrade RF, Resig S, Wentorf F, et al. The effects of grade III posterolateral knee complex injuries on anterior cruciate ligament graft force. A biomechanical analysis. Am J Sports Med 1999;27:469–75.
51. Kocher MS, Steadman JR, Briggs KK, et al. Relationships between objective assessment of ligament instability and subjective assessment of function after anterior cruciate ligament reconstruction. Am J Sports Med 2004;32:629–34.
52. Terry GC, Norwood LA, Hughston JC, et al. How iliotibial tract injuries of the knee combine with acute anterior cruciate ligament tears to influence abnormal anterior tibial displacement. Am J Sports Med 1993;21:55–60.
53. Norwood LA, Andrews JR, Meisterling RC, et al. Acute anterolateral rotary instability of the knee. J Bone Joint Surg Am 1979;61:704–9.
54. Hughston JC, Andrews JR, Cross MJ, et al. Classification of knee ligament instabilities. Part II. The lateral compartment. J Bone Joint Surg Am 1976;58:173–9.
55. Ellison AE. Distal iliotibial band transfer for anterolateral rotary instability of the knee. J Bone Joint Surg Am 1979;61:330–7.

56. Johnson LL. Lateral capsular ligament complex: anatomic and surgical considerations. Am J Sports Med 1979;7:156–60.

57. Claes S, Bartholomeeusen S, Bellemans J. High prevalence of anterolateral ligament injuries in magnetic resonance images of anterior cruciate ligament –injured knees. Acta Orthop Belg 2014;80:45–9.

58. Losee RE, Johnson TR, Southwick WO. Anterior subluxation of the lateral tibial plateau. J Bone Joint Surg Am 1978;60:1015–30.

59. Unverferth LJ, Bagenstose JE. Extra articular reconstructive surgery for combined anterolateral-anteromedial rotatory instability. Am J Sports Med 1979;7:34–9.

60. Muller W. The knee: form, function and ligament reconstruction. New York: Springer-Verlag; 1983. p. 253–7.

61. Noyes FR, Barber SD. The effect of an extra-articular procedure on allograft reconstructions for chronic ruptures of the anterior cruciate ligament. J Bone Joint Surg Am 1991;73:882–92.

62. Parsons EM, Gee AO, Spiekerman C, et al. The biomechanical function of the anterolateral ligament of the knee. Am J Sports Med 2015;43:669–74.

63. Rasmussen MT, Nitri M, Williams BT, et al. An in vitro robotic assessment of the anterolateral ligament, part 1: secondary role of the anterolateral, ligament in the setting of an anterior cruciate ligament injury. Am J Sports Med 2016;44:585–92.

64. Galway HR, MacIntosh DL. The lateral pivot shift: a symptom and sign of anterior cruciate ligament insufficiency. Clin Orthop Relat Res 1980;147:45–50.

65. Wroble RR, Grood ES, Cummings JS, et al. The role of the lateral extra articular restraints in the anterior cruciate ligament-deficient knee. Am J Sports Med 1993;21:257–63.

66. Tanaka M, Vyas D, Moloney G, et al. What does it take to have a high-grade pivot shift? Knee Surg Sports Traumatol Arthrosc 2012;20:147–52.

67. Bedi A, Musahl V, Lane C, et al. Lateral compartment translation predicts the grade of pivot shift: a cadaveric and clinical analysis. Knee Surg Sports Traumatol Arthrosc 2010;18:1269–76.

68. Musahl V, Citak M, O'Laughlin PF, et al. The effect of medial versus lateral meniscectomy on the stability of the anterior cruciate ligament-deficient knee. Am J Sports Med 2010;38:1591–7.

69. Helito CP, Helito PV, Costa HP, et al. Assessment of the anterolateral ligament of the knee by magnetic resonance imaging in acute injuries of the anterior cruciate ligament. Arthroscopy 2017;33:140–6.

70. Noyes FR, Huser LE, Levy MS. Rotational knee instability in ACL-deficient knees. J Bone Joint Surg Am 2017;99:305–14.

71. Nitri M, Rasmussen MT, Williams BT, et al. An in vitro robotic assessment of the anterolateral ligament, part 2: anterolateral ligament reconstruction combined with anterior cruciate ligament reconstruction. Am J Sports Med 2016;44:593–601.

72. Thein R, Boorman-Padgett J, Stone K, et al. Biomechanical assessment of the anterolateral ligament of the knee: a secondary restraint in simulated tests of the pivot shift and of anterior stability. J Bone Joint Surg Am 2016;98:937–43.

73. Diamantopoulos AP, Lorbach O, Paessler HH. Anterior cruciate ligament reconstruction revision: results in 107 patients. Am J Sports Med 2008;36:851–60.

74. Sonnery-Cottet B, Thaunat M, Freychet B, et al. Outcome of a combined anterior cruciate ligament an anterolateral reconstruction technique with a 2-year minimum follow up. Am J Sports Med 2015;43:1598–605.

75. Magnussen RA, Reinke EK, Huston LJ, et al. Effect of high-grade preoperative knee laxity on anterior cruciate ligament reconstruction outcomes. Am J Sports Med 2016;44:3077–82.

76. Greis PE, Steadman JR. Revision of failed prosthetic anterior cruciate ligament reconstruction. Clin Orthop Relat Res 1996;325:110–5.

77. Ahn JH, Lee YS, Ha HC. Comparison of revision surgery with primary anterior cruciate ligament reconstruction and outcome of revision surgery between different graft materials. Am J Sports Med 2008;36:1889–95.

78. Shelbourne KD, O'Shea JJ. Revision anterior cruciate ligament reconstruction using the bone-patellar tendon-bone graft. Instr Course Lect 2002;51:343–6.

79. Spindler KP, Kuhn JE, Freedman KB, et al. Anterior cruciate ligament reconstruction autograft choice: bone-tendon-bone versus hamstring: does it really matter? A systematic review. Am J Sports Med 2004;32:1986–95.

80. Wright RW, Gill CS, Chen L, et al. Outcome of revision anterior cruciate ligament reconstruction: a systematic review. J Bone Joint Surg Am 2012;94:531–6.

81. Wegrzyn J, Chouteau J, Philippot R, et al. Repeat revision of anterior cruciate ligament reconstruction: a retrospective review of management and outcome of 10 patients with an average 3-year follow up. Am J Sports Med 2009;37:77–85.

82. Magnussen RA. Third times a charm? Improving re-revision ACL reconstruction by addressing reasons for prior failures. Eur Orthop Traumatol 2012;3:55–60.

83. Matsumoto H, Seedhom BB. Treatment of the pivot-shift intraarticular versus extraarticular or combined procedures. A biomechanical study. Clin Orthop Relat Res 1994;299:298–304.

84. Mascarenhas R, Tranovich M, Karpie JC, et al. Patellar tendon anterior cruciate ligament reconstruction in the high demand patient: evaluation of autograft versus allograft reconstruction. Arthroscopy 2010;26(9Suppl):S58–66.

85. Ristanis S, Giakas G, Papageorgiou CD, et al. The effects of anterior cruciate ligament reconstruction on tibial rotation during pivoting after descending stairs. Knee Surg Sports Traumatol Arthrosc 2003;11:360–5.

86. Georgoulis AD, Ristanis S, Chouliaras V, et al. Tibial rotation is not restored after ACL reconstruction with a hamstring graft. Clin Orthop Relat Res 2007;454:89–94.

87. Hewison CE, Tran MN, Kaniki N, et al. Lateral extra articular tenodesis reduces rotational laxity when combined with anterior cruciate ligament reconstruction: a systematic review of the literature. Arthroscopy 2015;10:2022–34.

88. Biau DJ, Katsahian S, Kartus J, et al. Patellar tendon versus hamstring autografts for reconstructing the anterior cruciate ligament: a meta-analysis based on individual patient data. Am J Sports Med 2009;37:2470–8.

89. Blythe A, Tasker T, Zioupos P. ACL graft constructs: in –vitro fatigue testing highlights the occurrence of irrecoverable lengthening and the need for adequate (pre) conditioning to avert the recurrence of knee instability. Technol Health Care 2006;14:335–47.

90. Tomita F, Yasuda K, Mikami S, et al. Comparisons of intraosseous graft healing between doubled flexor tendon graft and the bone-patellar tendon-bone graft in anterior cruciate ligament reconstruction. Arthroscopy 2001;17:461–76.

91. Panni AS, Milano G, Luciana L, et al. Graft healing after anterior cruciate ligament reconstruction in rabbits. Clin Orthop Relat Res 1997;(343):203–12.

92. Draganich LF, Reider B, Ling M, et al. An in vitro study of an intraarticular and extra articular reconstruction in the anterior cruciate deficient knee. Am J Sports Med 1990;18:262–6.

93. Jackson DW, Grood ES, Goldstein JD, et al. A comparison of patellar tendon autograft and allograft used for anterior cruciate ligament reconstruction in the goat model. Am J Sports Med 1993;21:176–85.

94. Shino K, Gobbi A, Nakamura N, et al. How to handle a poorly placed femoral tunnel. In: Marx RG, editor. Revision ACL reconstruction: indications and technique. New York: Springer; 2014. p. 87–96.

95. Chouliaras V, Ristanis S, Moraiti C, et al. Effectiveness of reconstruction of the anterior cruciate ligament with quadrupled hamstrings and bone-patellar-bone autografts: an in vivo study comparing tibial internal-external rotation. Am J Sports Med 2007;35:189–96.

96. Draganich LF, Reider B, Miller PR. An in vitro study of the Muller anterolateral femorotibial ligament tenodesis in the anterior cruciate deficient knee. Am J Sports Med 1989;17:357–62.

Extra-Articular Plasty for Revision Anterior Cruciate Ligament Reconstruction

Panagiotis Ntagiopoulos, MD, PhD[a],*, David Dejour, MD[b]

KEYWORDS

- ACL reconstruction • ACL revision • Anterolateral ligament • Extra-articular plasty
- Lemaire

KEY POINTS

- Despite a well-performed anatomic anterior cruciate ligament (ACL) reconstruction, some patients continue to experience rotatory knee instability.
- In the setting of ACL rupture, the integrity of the anterolateral knee structures should always be evaluated.
- Although further studies are required, extra-articular lateral tenodesis at the time of ACL reconstruction may be beneficial in patients who have generalized ligamentous laxity, have a high-grade explosive pivot-shift test, participate in high-level sports, or are undergoing revision surgery and in chronic cases of damage to the anterolateral structures clearly evident clinically or radiographically.

INDICATIONS FOR EXTRA-ARTICULAR PLASTY

Recurrent or persistent laxity, in particular rotational laxity associated with a grossly positive pivot-shift test (PST), has been associated with the combined damage of the ACL and the anterolateral structures of the knee. Other investigators have also recorded probable evidence of damage of these structures along with ACL tears with the presence of a Segond fracture that results from avulsion of the iliotibial band (ITB) or the anterior oblique band of the lateral collateral ligament (LCL).[1–4] Further evidence of the gross instability after ACL and lateral structure damage is lateral tibial subluxation and the subsequent bone bruising observed on MRI.[5,6] As Dodds and colleagues[7] have recently reported, these anterolateral structures may not have been yet directly identified but probably act as secondary restraints of the PST, supplementing the primary role of the ACL in anteroposterior stability, with

Disclosure Statement: None of the authors have any conflict of interest.
[a] Hip & Knee Unit, Mediterraneo Hospital, 10 Ilias Street, Glyfada, Athens 16675, Greece;
[b] Orthopaedic Department, Lyon-Ortho-Clinic, Clinique de la Sauvegarde, Avenue Ben Gourion, Lyon 69009, France
* Corresponding author.
E-mail address: ntagiopoulos@hotmail.com

Clin Sports Med 37 (2018) 115–125
http://dx.doi.org/10.1016/j.csm.2017.07.009
0278-5919/18/© 2017 Elsevier Inc. All rights reserved.

sportsmed.theclinics.com

emphasis on rotatory stability. This rotatory laxity has been reported even after ACL reconstruction without failure of the ACL graft, suggesting that a single-bundle intra-articular reconstruction may not be sufficient to completely restore rotational knee stability in certain patients.[8]

The debate regarding combined injury to the ACL and anterolateral structures and the failure to provide rotatory stability in some patients has given rise to the strategy of combined intra-articular ACL reconstruction with extra-articular plasty.

The main arguments of the supporters of this procedure are as follows: (1) the evidence (discussed previously) of the additional structures being damaged in ACL tears favors the notion that additional structures need to be addressed at the time of ACL reconstruction; (2) the strong association of the anterolateral structures in controlling internal tibial rotation; and (3) the lateral extra-articular plasty is far from the center of the knee rotation and provides a greater lever arm for controlling PST and internal rotation than an intra-articular reconstruction.[7,9–11] The rationale behind extra-articular plasty is, therefore, to create a restraint to internal tibial rotation.

Investigators who favor supplementary extra-articular plasty with standard ACL reconstruction have reported reduced PST results[12,13] but the introduction of evidence-based inclusion criteria for any similar technique as a primary or a revision option is difficult and remains sporadic and empirically based.[7,11,13] In the authors' practice, extra-articular plasty is performed in conjunction with primary intra-articular ACL reconstruction in the following circumstances:

1. Challenging primary cases of gross PST recorded or patients with increased body mass index participating in high-level sports activities
2. Chronic cases of ACL injury where damage to the anterolateral structures of the knee is clinically or radiographically documented
3. Revision cases of ACL reconstruction, especially cases of previous graft placement that was anatomic and where rerupture was the result of minimal force
4. Patients with joint hyperlaxity

SURGICAL TECHNIQUES

There have been several techniques of extra-articular tenodesis described in the literature since the 1970s. MacIntosh and Darby[14] described a procedure where a 20-cm ITB strip was dissected, turned down to the Gerdy tubercle (GT), and then looped deep into the femoral condyle near the LCL. The Lemaire procedure involved the dissection of a 16-cm ITB strip, which was left attached to GT, passed under the LCL into a bone tunnel in the lateral femoral condyle, and then reattached to GT in a second bone tunnel.[15] The Ellison procedure was a modification of the MacIntosh procedure, where the ITB strip was detached from GT before being inserted in the femoral condyle.[16] Christel and Djian[17] described a less invasive modification of the original Lemaire procedure, where a shorter ITB strip was twisted 180° and inserted to the lateral femoral condyle. Losee and colleagues[2] published a technique where the ITB was slinged and reefed around the posterolateral corner of the knee. In contrast to previous techniques, in the late 1990s, Marcacci and colleagues[9] described a procedure of anterior cruciate ligament (ACL) reconstruction where a hamstrings graft was used both for intra-articular reconstruction and lateral tenodesis, through the over-the-top position. Several years later, Colombet[18] used a single-bundle hamstrings graft passed through a tibial and femoral tunnel and fixed to the GT to perform the combined reconstruction. Describing yet another technique, Neyret[19] proposed the combination of bone–patellar tendon–bone for intra-articular reconstruction and gracilis for extra-articular tenodesis.

Combined Anterior Cruciate Ligament Reconstruction and Lateral Plasty with Iliotibial Band (Senior Author's [Dr Dejour] Technique)

Extra-articular plasty or tenodesis is the authors' preferred surgical technique and involves the reconstruction of a lateral graft, as described by Lemaire[15] and by Christel and Djian.[17] The rationale of the procedure lies in the use of an ITB graft that passes under the LCL, which then acts as a pulley and is fixed to the femur near the lateral epicondyle. Usually, graft preparation for the extra-articular tenodesis follows the primary graft harvesting for ACL reconstruction (eg, patellar tendon, hamstrings, or quadriceps tendon) and is performed prior to arthroscopy.

1. The knee is prepared and draped in the 90° flexed position (**Fig. 1**).
2. Along the midline of the ITB, incise down to the GT (**Fig. 2**).
3. Divide the ITB to detach proximally a 10-mm wide and 80-mm long rectangular strip (**Fig. 3**).
4. Whipstitch the obtained graft (**Fig. 4**).
5. After ACL reconstruction, the rest of the procedure is continued with the knee held in neutral rotation and 120° of flexion (**Fig. 5**).
6. Identify the LCL and passed the graft under the LCL (**Fig. 6**).
7. The desired insertion point of the ITB graft lies 10-mm proximal and 10-mm posterior to the lateral epicondyle where the LCL is attached (**Fig. 7**).
8. Pass the ITB graft (**Fig. 8**A). Secure the sutures temporarily and tighten the construct (**Fig. 8**B). Fix the ITB graft under the LCL and into the femur in a separate tunnel than the intra-articular ACL graft (**Fig. 8**C).

PITFALLS AND COMPLICATIONS
Combined Anterior Cruciate Ligament Reconstruction and Lateral Plasty with Iliotibial Band

The addition of an extra-articular gesture in ACL reconstruction adds little difficulty to an already challenging procedure. Despite its popularity, ACL reconstruction remains technically demanding with a low threshold for complications. One of the complications of the extra-articular plasty is the improper placement of the additional femoral tunnel, and care must be taken to avoid converging with the intra-articular femoral tunnel because this leads to loss of primary fixation. Another drawback is the additional required skin and soft tissue exposure for the procedure along with donor-site morbidity of the ITB. Proper graft placement and tensioning are mandatory because

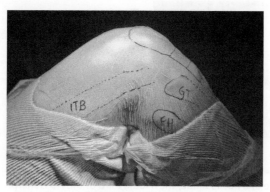

Fig. 1. The knee is prepared and draped in the 90° flexed position. Key anatomic landmarks for the procedure are ITB, GT, and the fibular head (FH).

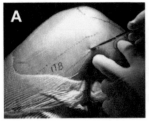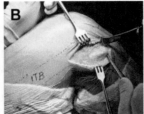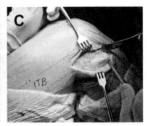

Fig. 2. Along the midline of the ITB and in line with the direction of its fibers, a 5-cm skin incision is performed down to the GT (*A*). Subcutaneous tissue is dissected to clearly visualize the ITB (*B*), especially its anterior and posterior borders (*C*).

malpositioning or over-tensioning the ITB graft leads to knee stiffness. A less aggressive rehabilitation program with a non–weight-bearing period of 3 weeks is advised to protect the extra-articular plasty.

Combined Anterior Cruciate Ligament Reconstruction and Lateral Plasty with Hamstrings

Graft rupture
Given that graft length is critical for the success of this technique, all possible events that could result in graft truncation at the time of harvest should be carefully avoided. Meticulous dissection of both gracilis and semitendinosus tendons from fascial attachments is mandatory to prevent premature amputation of the tendons when advancing the tendon stripper. If truncation of the graft occurs and 1 of the 2 tendons is shorter, the grafts can be sutured to each other and reconstruction can be performed according to the described technique. In most cases, the intra-articular graft is formed by 2 strands whereas the lateral plasty is inevitably formed by a biomechanically weaker single strand.

To gain an additional 1 cm or 2 cm in length, the distal attachment of the semitendinosus to the adjacent gracilis tendon can be dissected.

Another potential danger to graft integrity is the sharp edges of the tibial tunnel holes that may abrade or even cut the graft as it is being passed under tension. Therefore, before passing the graft through the tibial tunnel, the edges of the osseous tunnel should be accurately smoothened with a motorized shaver.

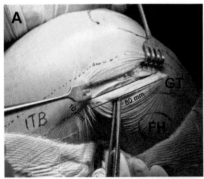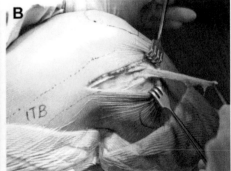

Fig. 3. With the use of a no. 15 blade, the middle third of the ITB is sharply divided to detach proximally a 10-mm wide and 80-mm long rectangular strip (*A*), while leaving its distal insertion attached to the GT (*B*). FH, fibular head.

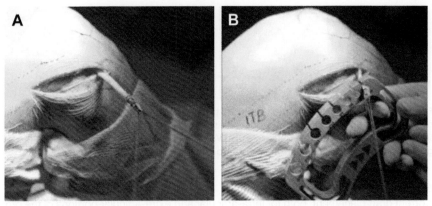

Fig. 4. The obtained graft is whip-stitched in a standard fashion (*A*) and sized (*B*).

Detachment of the distal insertion of the tendons from the anteromedial tibia can also be caused be caused by excessive graft tensioning. The graft, therefore, should be correctly tensioned with a progressive increase of force, avoiding sudden and forceful tensioning. In cases of detachment of the distal insertion of the tendons, both the strands of the distal end of the graft could be sutured together and the graft retrieved downward through the tibial tunnel and fixed with an interference screw or metal staple. At this point, the possibility of performing the lateral plasty depends from the remaining length of the graft.

Also, graft fixation with metal staples, especially at the lateral femoral cortex, could be a source of graft damage, because the barb of the metal staple coupled with high tension applied to the graft could produce a guillotine effect. To avoid this drawback, the staples should be firmly fixed in the bone cortex but not driven in too deeply. On the other hand, loose or insufficient fixation does not allow appropriate graft tensioning and almost certainly leads to failure of the reconstruction.

In cases of graft rupture, which do not allow for lateral plasty, the ACL reconstruction can be performed by maintaining only the intra-articular portion of the procedure, with an understanding of all the limitations inherent to a single-bundle, nonanatomic technique.

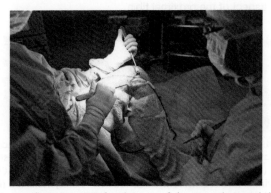

Fig. 5. The knee is now flexed in 120° for the rest of the procedure and the knee is held in neutral rotation.

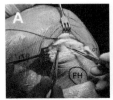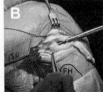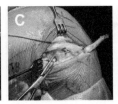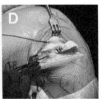

Fig. 6. This maneuver helps to easily identify the LCL that runs from the lateral femoral epicondyle to the fibular head (FH) (*A*). LCL is incised on its anterior and posterior borders and a small pulley is undermined with scissors (*B*). With the use of a curved Kelly clamp (*C*), the ITB graft is passed under the LCL from a distal to proximal direction (*D*).

Incorrect graft placement

Correct graft placement, both for intra-articular and extra-articular portions of the procedure, is imperative to obtain good outcomes and to avoid dangerous complications.

The execution of a tibial tunnel directed to the posteromedial part of ACL tibial insertion, coupled with the use of the over-the-top position, should guarantee the correct location of the graft. Nevertheless, in chronic cases, large osteophytes, especially on the medial edge of the lateral condyle, can obstruct the intercondylar notch, necessitating true notchplasty to avoid graft impingement. Any soft tissue in the posterior part of the roof that can obstruct the over-the-top position must be carefully removed as well.

The incorrect placement of the extra-articular plasty graft can produce excessive tension on the graft throughout knee range of motion, causing pain and joint stiffness. This can be avoided by fixing the graft in the isometric position. A small groove is first made in the lateral aspect of the femur, which allows graft anteriorization. To find the isometric point for distal fixation, the graft is cycled repeatedly, and graft tension is checked throughout the complete range of motion.

Iatrogenic injuries

Improper graft harvest may result in damage to important anatomic structures. The infrapatellar branches of the saphenous nerve can be harmed when performing the skin incision and tendon dissection; the risk is considered higher with harvest of bone–patellar tendon–bone compared with hamstrings. Performing an oblique rather than vertical incision theoretically reduces this risk. When the infrapatellar branches of the saphenous nerve are damaged, a patient may describe a patch of numbness on the anterolateral aspect of the proximal tibia.

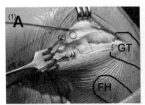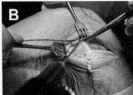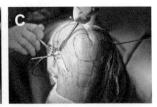

Fig. 7. The desired insertion point of the ITB graft lies 10-mm proximal and 10-mm posterior to the lateral epicondyle where the LCL is attached (*A*). In this case, the desired point is identified with a circle (2), while the pull-out sutures from the intra-articular ACL graft are visible (1). A Kirschner wire is inserted while the LCL course is closely followed (*B*). The Kirschner wire is carefully directed to not interfere with the intra-articular femoral ACL tunnel (*C*). FH, fibular head.

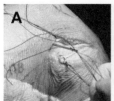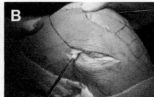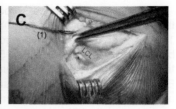

Fig. 8. A 6-mm cannulated drill is then used to gently create a unicortical tunnel of sufficient length to accommodate the full length of the ITB graft. Care is taken to not violate the far medial cortex. The ITB graft is then pulled medially into the new tunnel (A). An appropriately sized (7-mm) bioabsorbable interference screw is used for fixation of the graft while a Kocher clamp is used medially to secure the sutures temporarily and to tighten the construct (B). The final image of the extra-articular plasty shows the ITB graft passing under the LCL and fixed into the femur in a separate tunnel than the intra-articular ACL graft (1) (C).

When harvesting the gracilis and semitendinosus tendons, care should also be taken to not damage the superficial medial collateral ligament, because it lies immediately deep to the expansion of pes anserinus and should not be mistaken for it.

A more dangerous and harmful complication related to this technique is represented by injury of the popliteal artery when approaching the over-the-top position. Although this is a rare event, it should be considered a vascular emergency and its treatment is beyond the scope of this article.

LITERATURE RESULTS
Results of Extra-Articular Plasty in Anterior Cruciate Ligament Reconstruction Surgery

The extra-articular plasty was initially performed without concomitant intra-articular ACL reconstruction. Early results were not favorable mostly because of failure to restore anteroposterior stability and the development of postoperative lateral femoro-tibial degenerative changes.[2,20,21] Isolated extra-articular tenodesis was, however, soon abandoned due to donor site morbidity; the long rehabilitation protocol, which included a 2-month period of knee immobilization; and the concomitant development of less-invasive and cosmetically appealing all arthroscopic ACL reconstruction techniques.[7]

When extra-articular plasty was combined with intra-articular ACL reconstruction, the results were more encouraging. Dejour and colleagues[22] treated 148 patients with 11.5 years' follow-up using open intra-articular ACL reconstruction with bone–patellar tendon–bone autograft and extra-articular plasty using the Lemaire technique; 89% of patients were either satisfied or very satisfied with their results on subjective scoring. Using the same technique, Dejour and colleagues[23] also treated 251 cases of chronic ACL laxity and found that 83% of patients had good or excellent functional results. Jensen and colleagues[24] found no significant differences between intra-articular ACL reconstruction and additional extra-articular plasty, but they observed that extra-articular plasty reduced the subjective feeling of giving way in patients. Similarly, Noyes and Barber[25] and Lerat and colleagues[26] noted a significant increase in stability when extra-articular plasty was added to ACL reconstruction.

Successful results were also published by Ferretti and colleagues[27] in a study where the investigators, in the setting of revision ACL surgery, used an intra-articular recon-struction with a double-looped hamstrings graft and an extra-articular reconstruction, using a modification of the MacIntosh procedure.

Marcacci and colleagues[11] reported the long-term results of the nonanatomic over-the-top ACL reconstruction combined with lateral tenodesis using hamstrings graft. The investigators recommended this technique for primary ACL reconstruction because they found that 90% of 54 consecutive cases had good or excellent International Knee Documentation Committee scores at an average of 11 years' follow-up.[11] Bignozzi and colleagues[28] evaluated the results of the latter technique with computer-assisted navigation and found that the in vivo addition of an extra-articular procedure to single-bundle ACL reconstruction successfully controls tibial translation during the Lachman test and reduces anteroposterior laxity at 90° of flexion. Buda and colleagues[29] used the same nonanatomic over-the-top technique using allograft tendons for multiple-revision ACL reconstruction, reporting good or excellent results in 83% of patients, with 92% having a normal or nearly normal PST. Also, Trojani and colleagues[30] reported the results of ACL revision with additional lateral plasty, showing improved results in terms of stability and failure rate compared with isolated intra-articular reconstruction.

Although various techniques and graft choices have been described for lateral tenodesis procedures, most of these investigators agree that the point of femoral fixation is most critical.[7,10] The point of fixation should be located slightly posteriorly and proximally to the femoral insertion of the LCL.[31–33] In an effort to potentially identify this femoral insertion point more accurately, techniques that use intraoperative computer navigation have also been described.[18]

Comparison of Intra-Articular Anterior Cruciate Ligament Reconstruction with and Without Extra-Articular Plasty

A reasonable argument in favor of supplementary extra-articular plasty is that it provides additional protection of the intra-articular ACL reconstruction, especially in the early rehabilitation period. Even though the vitro study of extra-articular plasty has shown a decrease of up to 43% of the forces on the primary intra-articular construct,[34] the direct clinical value of the addition of extra-articular plasty has yet to be proved.[7] The few available studies that compare the 2 options produce contradicting results. Early reports showed no clear differences between intra-articular reconstruction with and without the addition of extra-articular plasty, suggesting no benefit from the supplementary procedure.[20,21,24,35–37] On the other hand, some investigators have noted benefits from the addition of extra-articular plasty, such as better PST control,[36] reduced tibial internal rotation, and produced higher constraint of lateral tibial displacement.[12,13,26,29] Monaco and colleagues[38] reported that the addition of extra-articular plasty significantly reduced internal tibial rotation at 30° of flexion compared with single-bundle or double-bundle ACL reconstruction. Zaffagnini and colleagues[39] compared single-bundle ACL reconstruction with and without extra-articular plasty and found superior results of the extra-articular plasty group in terms of subjective clinical findings and return-to-sport times. More recently, the same group compared double-bundle ACL reconstruction with combined single-bundle ACL reconstruction and extra-articular plasty. The latter resulted in better control of static knee laxity, reduced mediolateral instability in early flexion, and reduced rotatory instability at 90° of flexion.[13]

SUMMARY

With proper patient selection, the addition of an extra-articular plasty in the setting of primary or revision ACL reconstruction may lead to increased knee stability. Patients with gross ligamentous laxity or a preoperative explosive pivot-shift test should be carefully evaluated.

REFERENCES

1. Bull AM, Amis AA. The pivot-shift phenomenon: a clinical and biomechanical perspective. Knee 1998;5(5):141–58.
2. Losee RE, Johnson TR, Southwick WO. Anterior subluxation of the lateral tibial plateau. A diagnostic test and operative repair. J Bone Joint Surg Am 1978; 60(8):1015–30.
3. Norwood LA Jr, Andrews JR, Meisterling RC, et al. Acute anterolateral rotatory instability of the knee. J Bone Joint Surg Am 1979;61(5):704–9.
4. Campos JC, Chung CB, Lektrakul N, et al. Pathogenesis of the segond fracture: anatomic and MR imaging evidence of an iliotibial tract or anterior oblique band avulsion. Radiology 2001;219(2):381–6.
5. Delzell PB, Schils JP, Recht MP. Subtle fractures about the knee: innocuous-appearing yet indicative of significant internal derangement. AJR Am J Roentgenol 1996;167(3):699–703.
6. Tashiro Y, Okazaki K, Miura H, et al. Quantitative assessment of rotatory instability after anterior cruciate ligament reconstruction. Am J Sports Med 2009;37(5): 909–16.
7. Dodds AL, Gupte CM, Neyret P, et al. Extra-articular techniques in anterior cruciate ligament reconstruction: a literature review. J Bone Joint Surg Br 2011;93(11): 1440–8.
8. Tashman S, Collon D, Anderson K, et al. Abnormal rotational knee motion during running after anterior cruciate ligament reconstruction. Am J Sports Med 2004; 32(4):975–83.
9. Marcacci M, Zaffagnini S, Iacono F, et al. Arthroscopic intra- and extra-articular anterior cruciate ligament reconstruction with gracilis and semitendinosus tendons. Knee Surg Sports Traumatol Arthrosc 1998;6(2):68–75.
10. Marcacci M, Zaffagnini S, Marcheggiani Muccioli GM, et al. Arthroscopic intra- and extra-articular anterior cruciate ligament reconstruction with gracilis and semitendinosus tendons: a review. Curr Rev Musculoskelet Med 2011;4(2):73–7.
11. Marcacci M, Zaffagnini S, Giordano G, et al. Anterior cruciate ligament reconstruction associated with extra-articular tenodesis: a prospective clinical and radiographic evaluation with 10- to 13-year follow-up. Am J Sports Med 2009; 37(4):707–14.
12. Dejour D, Vanconcelos W, Bonin N, et al. Comparative study between mono-bundle bone-patellar tendon-bone, double-bundle hamstring and mono-bundle bone-patellar tendon-bone combined with a modified Lemaire extra-articular procedure in anterior cruciate ligament reconstruction. Int Orthop 2013;37(2):193–9.
13. Zaffagnini S, Signorelli C, Lopomo N, et al. Anatomic double-bundle and over-the-top single-bundle with additional extra-articular tenodesis: an in vivo quantitative assessment of knee laxity in two different ACL reconstructions. Knee Surg Sports Traumatol Arthrosc 2012;20(1):153–9.
14. Macintosh DL, Darby JA. Lateral substitution reconstruction. Proceedings of the Canadian Orthopaedic Association. J Bone Joint Surg Br 1976;(58):142.
15. Lemaire M. Chronic knee instability. Technics and results of ligament plasty in sports injuries. J Chir (Paris) 1975;110(4):281–94 [in French].
16. Ellison AE. Distal iliotibial-band transfer for anterolateral rotatory instability of the knee. J Bone Joint Surg Am 1979;61(3):330–7.
17. Christel P, Djian P. Anterio-lateral extra-articular tenodesis of the knee using a short strip of fascia lata. Rev Chir Orthop Reparatrice Appar Mot 2002;88(5): 508–13 [in French].

18. Colombet PD. Navigated intra-articular ACL reconstruction with additional extra-articular tenodesis using the same hamstring graft. Knee Surg Sports Traumatol Arthrosc 2011;19(3):384–9.
19. Duthon VB, Magnussen RA, Servien E, et al. ACL reconstruction and extra-articular tenodesis. Clin Sports Med 2013;32(1):141–53.
20. Roth JH, Kennedy JC, Lockstadt H, et al. Intra-articular reconstruction of the anterior cruciate ligament with and without extra-articular supplementation by transfer of the biceps femoris tendon. J Bone Joint Surg Am 1987;69(2):275–8.
21. Strum GM, Fox JM, Ferkel RD, et al. Intraarticular versus intraarticular and extra-articular reconstruction for chronic anterior cruciate ligament instability. Clin Orthop Relat Res 1989;(245):188–98.
22. Dejour H, Dejour D, Ait Si Selmi T. Chronic anterior laxity of the knee treated with free patellar graft and extra-articular lateral plasty: 10-year follow-up of 148 cases. Rev Chir Orthop Reparatrice Appar Mot 1999;85(8):777–89 [in French].
23. Dejour H, Walch G, Neyret P, et al. Results of surgically treated chronic anterior laxities. Apropos of 251 cases reviewed with a minimum follow-up of 3 years. Rev Chir Orthop Reparatrice Appar Mot 1988;74(7):622–36 [in French].
24. Jensen JE, Slocum DB, Larson RL, et al. Reconstruction procedures for anterior cruciate ligament insufficiency: a computer analysis of clinical results. Am J Sports Med 1983;11(4):240–8.
25. Noyes FR, Barber SD. The effect of an extra-articular procedure on allograft reconstructions for chronic ruptures of the anterior cruciate ligament. J Bone Joint Surg Am 1991;73(6):882–92.
26. Lerat JL, Chotel F, Besse JL, et al. The results after 10-16 years of the treatment of chronic anterior laxity of the knee using reconstruction of the anterior cruciate ligament with a patellar tendon graft combined with an external extra-articular reconstruction. Rev Chir Orthop Reparatrice Appar Mot 1998;84(8):712–27 [in French].
27. Ferretti A, Conteduca F, Monaco E, et al. Revision anterior cruciate ligament reconstruction with doubled semitendinosus and gracilis tendons and lateral extra-articular reconstruction. J Bone Joint Surg Am 2006;88(11):2373–9.
28. Bignozzi S, Zaffagnini S, Lopomo N, et al. Does a lateral plasty control coupled translation during antero-posterior stress in single-bundle ACL reconstruction? An in vivo study. Knee Surg Sports Traumatol Arthrosc 2009;17(1):65–70.
29. Buda R, Ruffilli A, Di Caprio F, et al. Allograft salvage procedure in multiple-revision anterior cruciate ligament reconstruction. Am J Sports Med 2013;41(2):402–10.
30. Trojani C, Beaufils P, Burdin G, et al. Revision ACL reconstruction: influence of a lateral tenodesis. Knee Surg Sports Traumatol Arthrosc 2012;20(8):1565–70.
31. Bylski-Austrow DI, Grood ES, Hefzy MS, et al. Anterior cruciate ligament replacements: a mechanical study of femoral attachment location, flexion angle at tensioning, and initial tension. J Orthop Res 1990;8(4):522–31.
32. Draganich LF, Hsieh YF, Reider B. Iliotibial band tenodesis: a new strategy for attachment. Am J Sports Med 1995;23(2):186–95.
33. Krackow KA, Brooks RL. Optimization of knee ligament position for lateral extra-articular reconstruction. Am J Sports Med 1983;11(5):293–302.
34. Engebretsen L, Lew WD, Lewis JL, et al. The effect of an iliotibial tenodesis on intraarticular graft forces and knee joint motion. Am J Sports Med 1990;18(2):169–76.
35. Amis AA, Scammell BE. Biomechanics of intra-articular and extra-articular reconstruction of the anterior cruciate ligament. J Bone Joint Surg Br 1993;75(5):812–7.

36. Giraud B, Besse JL, Cladiere F, et al. Intra-articular reconstruction of the anterior cruciate ligament with and without extra-articular supplementation by quadricipital tendon plasty: seven-year follow-up. Rev Chir Orthop Reparatrice Appar Mot 2006;92(8):788–97 [in French].
37. O'Brien SJ, Warren RF, Pavlov H, et al. Reconstruction of the chronically insufficient anterior cruciate ligament with the central third of the patellar ligament. J Bone Joint Surg Am 1991;73(2):278–86.
38. Monaco E, Labianca L, Conteduca F, et al. Double bundle or single bundle plus extraarticular tenodesis in ACL reconstruction? A CAOS study. Knee Surg Sports Traumatol Arthrosc 2007;15(10):1168–74.
39. Zaffagnini S, Marcacci M, Lo Presti M, et al. Prospective and randomized evaluation of ACL reconstruction with three techniques: a clinical and radiographic evaluation at 5 years follow-up. Knee Surg Sports Traumatol Arthrosc 2006;14(11):1060–9.

The Influence of Tibial and Femoral Bone Morphology on Knee Kinematics in the Anterior Cruciate Ligament Injured Knee

Drew Lansdown, MD, Chunbong Benjamin Ma, MD*

KEYWORDS

- Bone morphology • Anterior cruciate ligament injuries • Knee kinematics
- Tibial slope • Intercondylar notch shape

KEY POINTS

- Morphologic variations in the tibia and femur influence the kinematics of the knee and contribute to risk of anterior cruciate ligament (ACL) injury as well as function of the knee after injury and after surgical reconstruction.
- Increases in posterior tibial slope result in increased forces across the ACL and increased anterior tibial translation.
- A shallow medial tibial plateau and lower volume of the medial tibial eminence lead to less bony congruity and place greater demand on ligamentous restraint in the knee.
- A dome-shaped intercondylar notch and spherical femoral condyles have been linked to worse patient-reported knee stability scores after ACL injury.

INTRODUCTION

Anterior cruciate ligament (ACL) injuries occur frequently in young, active patients and are a common cause of disability in this group of patients. ACL injuries place patients at risk for the development of posttraumatic osteoarthritis, further contributing to limited function of the injured knee.[1] There are approximately 250,000 ACL injuries in the United States alone each year, with 175,000 of these patients electing to undergo surgical reconstruction.[2,3]

The stability of the knee after an isolated ACL injury is variable, with a subset of patients reporting minimal instability whereas others face profound limitations from this

Department of Orthopaedic Surgery, University of California, San Francisco, 1500 Owens Street, Suite 186, San Francisco, CA 94158, USA
* Corresponding author.
E-mail address: maben@ucsf.edu

Clin Sports Med 37 (2018) 127–136
http://dx.doi.org/10.1016/j.csm.2017.07.012
0278-5919/18/© 2017 Elsevier Inc. All rights reserved.

sportsmed.theclinics.com

injury.[4,5] Multiple factors contribute to knee stability both after ACL injury and after ACL reconstruction. There has been renewed interest recently in the role of additional extra-articular procedures in the setting of failed reconstruction or patients with increased preoperative knee laxity.[6] Clear indications regarding utilization of these procedures remains unclear. One factor that contributes to knee kinematics that determines this spectrum of instability, from patients who may cope with an isolated ACL injury to those who may require a lateral extra-articular reconstruction to eliminate a pivot shift phenomenon, may be the bony geometry of the knee. There is a need to clarify which patients will benefit most from surgical reconstruction and from supplemental procedures in addition to ACL reconstruction, and there is potential that the anatomic differences with regard to bone shape may be an important factor in determining appropriate treatment recommendations. The purpose of this article is to review the current evidence on the contribution of tibial and femoral bone morphology to knee kinematics.

TIBIAL BONE MORPHOLOGY

The articular geometry of the tibial plateau influences the stability of the knee after ACL injury and changes the forces transmitted through the cruciate ligaments. The lateral plateau is convex compared with the concave medial plateau with increased congruity with its femoral condyle, which leads to more translational motion at the lateral side of the knee.[7,8] The posterior slope of the knee also contributes to the magnitude of the pivot shift, because the femoral condyle can translate more with an increased posterior tibial slope.[9] Increased motion at the anterior lateral tibial plateau may be responsible for tibial subluxation at the initiation of knee flexion[10] and may be associated with the severity of the pivot shift.[11]

Marouane and colleagues[12] investigated the effects of varying the posterior tibial slope on knee kinematics and forces across the ACL. The kinematic changes were calculated through finite element modeling of the normal gait cycle. With increases in posterior tibial slope, the anterior tibial translation increased, whereas decreased anterior tibial translation was observed with a lower tibial slope. The force across the ACL increased from 181 N to 317 N with a 5° increase in posterior tibial slope and to 460 N with a 10° slope increase. This force decreased to 102 N by decreasing posterior slope by 5°, and the ACL was offloaded completely by decreasing posterior slope by 10°. The observed effects would likely be further increased with greater external loads through larger muscle activation forces. Multiple cadaveric studies have also demonstrated that an increase in the tibial slope results in increasingly anterior resting position of the tibia relative to the femur.[13–15]

Shelburne and colleagues[16] reported how posterior tibial slope effected the forces across the cruciate ligaments and knee-joint loading in a finite element model during standing, squatting, and walking. For all positions, there was a linear relationship between the posterior tibial slope and cruciate ligament forces, and tibial shear force as well as anterior tibial translation. Tibial shear force, which is determined by the posterior tibial slope, has been shown to determine the forces across the cruciate ligaments.[17,18] Therefore, the shape of the proximal tibia is a strong contributor to forces across the ACL and kinematics of the knee.

Tibial slope is the most frequently reported bone shape feature implicated in ACL injury and risk of failure after ACL reconstruction. Dejour and Bonnin[19] radiographically measured anterior tibial translation on the lateral standing, bent-knee radiographs of 281 patients with chronic ACL injuries. Posterior tibial slope is measured on radiographs, first defining the longitudinal axis of the tibia with 2 points equidistant between the anterior and posterior tibial cortices just distal to the tibial tubercle and a second 10-cm distal to this first point (**Fig. 1**). A line perpendicular to this is drawn at the joint line, and the angle between this line and a line along the tibial plateau defines the tibial slope. The amount of anterior tibial translation was directly and significantly correlated with the magnitude of the posterior tibial slope, with 6 mm of anterior tibial translation observed for each 10° that tibial slope increased. This study is in agreement with the cadaveric and modeling studies that show the influence of tibial slope on knee kinematics and force across the ACL.

Multiple clinical case-control studies have found increased posterior tibial slope as a risk factor for sustaining a noncontact ACL injury. Brandon and colleagues[11] found the posterior tibial slope higher for both female patients (12.6° vs 8.6°; $P<.001$) and male patients (10.8° vs 8.4°; $P<.001$) with ACL injuries relative to patients with patellofemoral pain. Additionally, among patients with ACL injuries, those with a more severe pivot-shift grade had increased posterior tibial slope relative to those with a lower-grade pivot shift (11.1° vs 9.2°; $P = .03$). Other case-control studies have identified increased posterior slope as a risk factor for ACL injury in both male patients and female patients[20] or female patients alone.[21]

The effects of posterior tibial slope also seem different between the medial and lateral sides of the knee, with the lateral side more consistently having a larger impact on knee kinematics. Stijak and colleagues[22] reported increased lateral tibial slope in patients with ACL injuries relative to control patients (7.5° vs 4.4°) whereas there was no increase with the slope of the medial plateau (5.2° vs 6.6°). Other case-control studies have

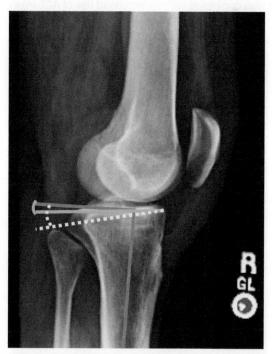

Fig. 1. The posterior tibial slope is defined on the lateral radiograph by measuring the angle between the diaphyseal axis (*blue line*) of the tibia and the tibial plateau (*green line*). An increased posterior tibial slope (*dotted yellow line*) is associated with increased anterior tibial translation and increased force across the ACL.

found that both the medial and lateral plateaus[23] or just the lateral plateau in men[24] showed increased posterior slope in patients with ACL injuries. In a recent meta-analysis of studies evaluating the impact of tibial slope on ACL injury, Zeng and colleagues[25] found that both the medial and lateral slope seemed associated with increasing the risk of ACL injury. The evidence for lateral tibial plateau slope as a risk factor for ACL injury was overall stronger and more consistent. These studies suggest the slope, particularly of the lateral tibial plateau, places patients at risk for ACL injuries, likely through the mechanism of increased translation of the lateral tibia and greater stress across the ACL.

The depth of the medial tibial plateau has also been implicated in contributing to the risk of ACL injury. The medial plateau has a concave shape that allows for inherent congruity with the medial femoral condyle and is more constrained relative to the convex lateral plateau. Hashemi and colleagues[23] measured the depth of the medial tibial plateau on MRI for 49 patients with ACL injuries and 55 subjects without ACL injury. A shallower medial tibial plateau was noted in patients with ACL injuries (**Fig. 2**). This finding suggests that patients with ACL injury may have bone shape features, such as a shallow medial tibial plateau, that predispose to ligamentous injury, which may help identify patients who may benefit from additional procedures in addition to ACL reconstruction, although this hypothesis needs further clinical and biomechanical testing.

The volume of the medial tibial spine was identified by Sturnick and colleagues[26] as a potential risk factor for ACL injury. MRI was used to calculate this volume for patients with and without ACL injuries. Among male patients specifically, a lower volume of the medial tibial spine was correlated with an increased risk of ACL injury. Through normal

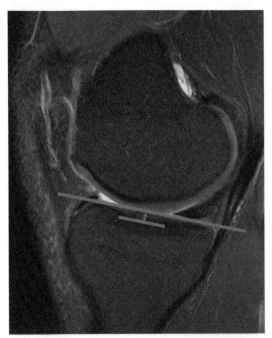

Fig. 2. The depth of the medial plateau was shown by Hashemi and colleagues[23] as associated with the risk of ACL injury. A shallow medial tibial plateau, measured as shown on a sagittal MRI, may be associated with less articular congruity and greater risk of ACL injury.

knee range of motion, the tibial spines have some articulation with the femoral condyles. Motion of the knee may vary with different shapes of the tibial spines, and patients with smaller spines may continue to have abnormal knee kinematics even after ACL reconstruction.

FEMORAL BONE MORPHOLOGY

Variations in femoral morphology have also been reported to influence knee kinematics. Differences in intercondylar notch morphology are the most commonly reported bone feature on the femoral side to be associated with ACL injury. Eggerding and colleagues[27] followed 257 patients prospectively after ACL injury to determine if morphologic features identified on radiographs could predict International Knee Documentation Committee (IKDC) knee stability scores. Statistical shape modeling, which is an unbiased method for determining unique shape features common within a group of patients, was used to explore bony geometry on lateral and 45° bent-knee posteroanterior radiographs. A pyramid-shaped intercondylar notch was associated with higher IKDC scores 2 years after injury compared with patients with dome-shaped intercondylar notches (**Fig. 3**). This pyramid shape of the intercondylar notch was theorized to lead to a more intrinsically stable joint that relies less on ligamentous function. As demonstrated in this study, certain bone features may help in predicting which patients will tolerate an ACL deficiency state whereas others may continue to have instability after anatomic ACL reconstruction.

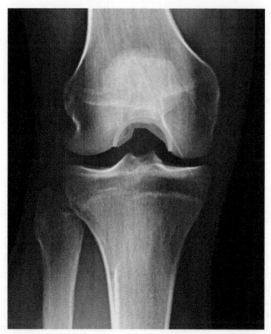

Fig. 3. The intercondylar notch shape has been implicated as a risk factor for ACL injury. A pyramidal notch shape, present in this patient and outlined in blue, may lead to greater bony congruity of the knee and was found to be associated with better knee stability scores at 2 years after nonoperatively treated ACL injuries compared with a dome-shaped notch, outlined in green.

A

Tibial Slope

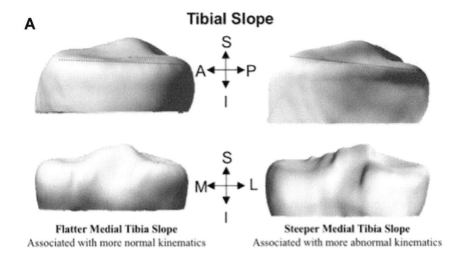

Flatter Medial Tibia Slope
Associated with more normal kinematics

Steeper Medial Tibia Slope
Associated with more abnormal kinematics

B

Sphericity of Medial Femoral Condyle

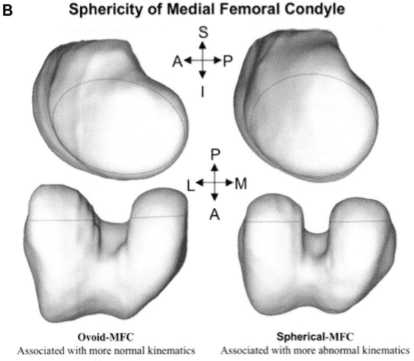

Ovoid-MFC
Associated with more normal kinematics

Spherical-MFC
Associated with more abnormal kinematics

Fig. 4. Two shapes identified through statistical shape modeling that were identified as associated with abnormal post–ACL injury and postreconstruction knee kinematics were the slope of the medial tibial plateau and the sphericity of the medial femoral condyle. A flatter medial tibial slope (*A*) was associated with knee kinematics that were more similar to the patient's contralateral knee, whereas a steeper medial tibial slope was associated with greater anterior tibial translation. A more ovoid-shaped medial femoral condyle (*B*) was associated with more similar kinematics compared with the patient's contralateral knee, whereas a more spherical shaped medial femoral condyle was associated with greater anterior tibial translation. A, anterior; I, inferior; L, lateral; M, medial; MFC, medial femoral condyle; P, posterior; S, superior.

Fridén and colleagues[28] also investigated for potential bony factors that contribute to subjective instability after ACL injury. A series of 100 patients with ACL injuries and limited activity levels were followed for 5 years. There were 16 patients who elected to undergo ACL reconstruction, and a more spherical shape of the femoral condyles was correlated with patients who had failed nonoperative treatment. Differences in the shape of the femoral condyles may lead to variability in knee kinematics and differential injury risk and subjective stability.

3-D SHAPE STUDY

The authors' group has used 3-D statistical shape modeling with MRI-based knee kinematics to correlate the relationship between specific bone morphologic features and postsurgical knee kinematics after ACL reconstruction.[29] There was wide variation in the postreconstruction anterior tibial translation of the reconstructed knee compared with a patient's normal, contralateral knee in patients with isolated ACL injuries, and the amount of both postinjury and postreconstruction anterior tibial translation was associated with morphologic features of both the tibia and femur. Greater slope of the medial tibial plateau (**Fig. 4**A), a more spherical medial femoral condyle (see **Fig. 4**B), and increased length of the lateral tibial plateau were all associated with abnormal postinjury and postsurgical knee kinematics. A shorter medial tibial plateau, like that observed by Hashemi and colleagues[23] was also associated with abnormal postsurgical knee kinematics. The findings in this prospective study with 3-D imaging and sophisticated shape determination algorithms corroborate many of the findings identified in previous retrospective studies, given further strength to the relationships proposed between bone morphology and knee kinematics.

SURGICAL CONSIDERATIONS

Posterior tibial slope is one factor that may be altered surgically. Dejour and colleagues[30] reported on a series of 9 patients who were treated with second-time revision ACL reconstruction. In this series, the patients were also treated with a deflexion tibial osteotomy, decreasing the mean posterior tibial slope of the group from 13.2° to 4.4°. With this bony correction, the anterior tibial translation decreased from 11.7 mm prior to surgery to 4.3 mm after reconstruction. These results highlight the importance

Table 1
Bone shape features and their relationship to knee kinematics

Bone Shape Feature	Correlation With Knee Kinematics
Posterior-inferior tibial slope	Increasing posterior-inferior tibial slope is correlated with increased anterior tibial translation and force across ACL.
Depth of medial tibial plateau	Decreasing depth of medial tibial plateau is associated with decreased bony congruity in the medial compartment.
Volume of medial tibial eminence	Decreased volume of medial tibial eminence is associated with decreased contact area.
Notch shape	Pyramidal notch shape may lead to more intrinsically stable knee whereas dome-shaped notch may be more dependent on ACL for stability.
Sphericity of femoral condyles	More spherical femoral condyles, particularly medial, associated with abnormal knee kinematics after surgery and after ACL reconstruction and increased risk of symptomatic instability.

of considering bone morphology, especially when contemplating revision ACL reconstruction. Correction of an increased posterior tibial slope should be strongly considered in the setting of a failed ACL reconstruction and 13° or more of posterior tibial slope. Many of the other bony features discussed in this article that have an impact on knee kinematics and lead to an increased ACL injury risk may not be modifiable. These findings, however, may still have great utility when dealing with patients at risk for ACL injury, after primary ACL injury or after failed reconstruction, and may prove to be important in clarifying indications for extra-articular reconstructive procedures.

SUMMARY

Future clinical and biomechanical studies should evaluate how bone morphology may contribute to knee kinematics after isolated ACL reconstruction or combined with lateral extra-articular reconstruction procedures. Further studies using 3-D imaging and statistical shape modeling will aide in clarifying the role of various bone features in knee kinematics (**Table 1**). Patients with certain tibial and femoral morphologic features may remain at risk for ACL injury even after an anatomic ligament reconstruction due to the articular geometry that may increase anterior tibial translation and stress across the ACL. The patients with the specific bone features described in this article will benefit from further evaluation as to the optimal surgical reconstructive techniques and methods to achieve a stable and functional knee.

REFERENCES

1. Lohmander LS, Östenberg A, Englund M, et al. High prevalence of knee osteoarthritis, pain, and functional limitations in female soccer players twelve years after anterior cruciate ligament injury. Arthritis Rheum 2004;50(10):3145–52.
2. Hewett TE, Myer GD, Ford KR, et al. Mechanisms, prediction & prevention of ACL injuries: cut risk with 3 sharpened & validated tools. J Orthop Res 2016;34(11): 1843–55.
3. Spindler KP, Wright RW. Anterior cruciate ligament tear. N Engl J Med 2008; 359(20):2135–42.
4. Barrance PJ, Williams GN, Snyder-Mackler L, et al. Altered knee kinematics in ACL-deficient non-copers: a comparison using dynamic MRI. J Orthop Res 2006;24(2):132–40.
5. Barrance PJ, Williams GN, Snyder-Mackler L, et al. Do ACL-injured copers exhibit differences in knee kinematics?: an MRI study. Clin Orthop Relat Res 2007;454: 74–80.
6. Magnussen RA, Reinke EK, Huston LJ, et al. Effect of high-grade preoperative knee laxity on anterior cruciate ligament reconstruction outcomes. Am J Sports Med 2016;44(12):3077–82.
7. Amis AA. Anterolateral knee biomechanics. Knee Surg Sports Traumatol Arthrosc 2017;25(4):1015–23.
8. Mahfouz MR, Komistek RD, Dennis DA, et al. In vivo assessment of the kinematics in normal and anterior cruciate ligament-deficient knees. J Bone Joint Surg Am 2004;86(Suppl 2):56–61.
9. østgaard SE, Helmig P, Nielsen S, et al. Anterolateral instability in the anterior cruciate ligament deficient knee: a cadaver study. Acta Orthop Scand 1991; 62(1):4–8.

10. Bull A, Earnshaw P, Smith A, et al. Intraoperative measurement of knee kinematics in reconstruction of the anterior cruciate ligament. J Bone Joint Surg Br 2002; 84(7):1075–81.

11. Brandon ML, Haynes PT, Bonamo JR, et al. The association between posterior-inferior tibial slope and anterior cruciate ligament insufficiency. Arthroscopy 2006;22(8):894–9.

12. Marouane H, Shirazi-Adl A, Hashemi J. Quantification of the role of tibial posterior slope in knee joint mechanics and ACL force in simulated gait. J Biomech 2015; 48(10):1899–905.

13. Agneskirchner J, Hurschler C, Stukenborg-Colsman C, et al. Effect of high tibial flexion osteotomy on cartilage pressure and joint kinematics: a biomechanical study in human cadaveric knees. Arch Orthop Trauma Surg 2004;124(9):575–84.

14. Rodner CM, Adams DJ, Diaz-Doran V, et al. Medial opening wedge tibial osteotomy and the sagittal plane the effect of increasing tibial slope on tibiofemoral contact pressure. Am J Sports Med 2006;34(9):1431–41.

15. Giffin JR, Vogrin TM, Zantop T, et al. Effects of increasing tibial slope on the biomechanics of the knee. Am J Sports Med 2004;32(2):376–82.

16. Shelburne KB, Kim HJ, Sterett WI, et al. Effect of posterior tibial slope on knee biomechanics during functional activity. J Orthop Res 2011;29(2):223–31.

17. Pandy MG, Shelburne KB. Dependence of cruciate-ligament loading on muscle forces and external load. J Biomech 1997;30(10):1015–24.

18. Shelburne KB, Pandy MG, Anderson FC, et al. Pattern of anterior cruciate ligament force in normal walking. J Biomech 2004;37(6):797–805.

19. Dejour H, Bonnin M. Tibial translation after anterior cruciate ligament rupture. Two radiological tests compared. J Bone Joint Surg Br 1994;76-B(5):745–9.

20. Todd MS, Lalliss S, Garcia ES. The relationship between posterior tibial slope and anterior cruciate ligament injuries. Am J Sports Med 2010;38(1):63–7.

21. Hohmann E, Bryant A, Reaburn P, et al. Is there a correlation between posterior tibial slope and non-contact anterior cruciate ligament injuries? Knee Surg Sports Traumatol Arthrosc 2011;19(1):109–14.

22. Stijak L, Herzog RF, Schai P. Is there an influence of the tibial slope of the lateral condyle on the ACL lesion? Knee Surg Sports Traumatol Arthrosc 2008;16(2): 112–7.

23. Hashemi J, Chandrashekar N, Mansouri H, et al. Shallow medial tibial plateau and steep medial and lateral tibial slopes new risk factors for anterior cruciate ligament injuries. Am J Sports Med 2010;38(1):54–62.

24. Bisson LJ, Gurske-DePerio J. Axial and sagittal knee geometry as a risk factor for noncontact anterior cruciate ligament tear: a case-control study. Arthroscopy 2010;26(7):901–6.

25. Zeng C, Cheng L, Wei J, et al. The influence of the tibial plateau slopes on injury of the anterior cruciate ligament: a meta-analysis. Knee Surg Sports Traumatol Arthrosc 2014;22(1):53–65.

26. Sturnick DR, Argentieri EC, Vacek PM, et al. A decreased volume of the medial tibial spine is associated with an increased risk of suffering an anterior cruciate ligament injury for males but not females. J Orthop Res 2014;32(11):1451–7.

27. Eggerding V, van Kuijk K, van Meer B, et al. Knee shape might predict clinical outcome after an anterior cruciate ligament rupture. Bone Joint J 2014;96(6): 737–42.

28. Fridén T, Jonsson A, Erlandsson T, et al. Effect of femoral condyle configuration on disability after an anterior cruciate ligament rupture: 100 patients followed for 5 years. Acta Orthop Scand 1993;64(5):571–4.

29. Lansdown DA, Pedoia V, Zaid M, et al. Variations in knee kinematics after ACL injury and after reconstruction are correlated with bone shape differences. Clin Orthop Relat Res 2017. http://dx.doi.org/10.1007/s11999-017-5368-8.
30. Dejour D, Saffarini M, Demey G, et al. Tibial slope correction combined with second revision ACL produces good knee stability and prevents graft rupture. Knee Surg Sports Traumatol Arthrosc 2015;23(10):2846–52.

What Is the State of the Evidence in Anterolateral Ligament Research?

Paul A. Moroz, MD (Cand)[a], Emily E. Quick, MD (Cand)[b],
Nolan S. Horner, MD[b], Andrew Duong, MSc[c],
Nicole Simunovic, MSc[d], Olufemi R. Ayeni, MD, MSc, FRCSC[e],*

KEYWORDS

- Anterolateral ligament • Short lateral ligament
- Capsulo-osseous layer of the iliotibial band • Mid-third lateral capsular ligament
- Anterior band of the lateral collateral ligament • Anterior oblique band

KEY POINTS

- The anterolateral ligament (ALL) of the knee is a capsular structure that runs from the lateral femoral epicondyle to the lateral tibial plateau and has been the subject of recent renewed academic interest.
- Presently available literature on the ALL is limited in both volume and quality.
- Most research on the ALL consists of biomechanical, cadaveric, or radiographic studies whose primary goals are establishing fundamental biomechanical, anatomic, and/or radiographic properties of the ALL.
- There are few studies to date pertaining to the diagnosis, therapy, prevalence, or prognosis of injury to the ALL.
- Analysis of current ALL research suggests a need to increase the volume of high quality clinical and radiographic studies to expand knowledge regarding the role of the ALL in ligamentous knee injury and elucidate the optimal imaging technique, for both the intact and injured ALL.

Disclosures: There are no commercial or financial conflicts of interest.
[a] Faculty of Medicine, University of British Columbia, 2350Health Sciences Mall, Vancouver, British Columbia V6T 1Z3, Canada; [b] Department of Medicine, Michael G. DeGroote School of Medicine, McMaster University, 1280 Main Street West, Hamilton, Ontario L8S 4K1, Canada; [c] Division of Orthopaedic Surgery, Department of Surgery, McMaster University, 1200 Main Street West, Hamilton, Ontario L8N 3Z5, Canada; [d] Department of Clinical Epidemiology and Biostatistics, Centre for Evidence-Based Orthopaedics, McMaster University, 1280 Main Street West, Hamilton, Ontario L8S4L8, Canada; [e] Department of Clinical Epidemiology and Biostatistics, Centre for Evidence-Based Orthopaedics, McMaster University, McMaster University Medical Center, 1200 Main Street West, Room 4E15, Hamilton, Ontario L8N 3Z5, Canada
* Corresponding author.
E-mail address: femiayeni@gmail.com

Clin Sports Med 37 (2018) 137–159
http://dx.doi.org/10.1016/j.csm.2017.07.013
0278-5919/18/© 2017 Elsevier Inc. All rights reserved.

INTRODUCTION

The anterolateral ligament (ALL) of the knee is a capsular structure that runs from the lateral femoral epicondyle to the lateral tibial plateau.[1] This structure was initially described by Segond[2] in 1879 as a pearly fibrous thickening of the lateral knee capsule that emerged from the iliotibial band. Since Segond,[2] several investigators have described what is understood to be the ALL and imparted a variety of names to this ligament. Previous terms and structures related to the ALL include anterolateral capsule, capsulo-osseous layer of the iliotibial band, mid-third lateral capsular ligament, anterior band of the lateral collateral ligament, and anterior oblique band.[3–7] The term "anterolateral ligament," coined by Vieira and colleagues[8] in 2012, appears to have become the common term used in recent literature.

Since its discovery, the ALL has been largely overlooked, and research into this structure throughout the twentieth century was limited. The recent popularity of anterior cruciate ligament (ACL) reconstruction has brought attention to the ALL and contributed to an expansion of research into this structure. A systematic review conducted by Van der Watt and colleagues,[1] found that the ALL was a distinct entity present in 96% of examined specimens, although prevalence across individual studies varied considerably. Several biomechanical studies suggest that the ALL contributes to rotary knee stability and thus playing a role in the pivot shift phenomenon.[9,10] Proposed indications for combined ACL and ALL reconstruction or lateral extra-articular tenodesis include ACL tear with grade 3 + pivot shift, chronic ACL lesion, persistent pivot shift in the setting of multiple revision ACL reconstructions, radiographic lateral femoral notch sign, involvement in pivoting sports, and significant instability following ACL reconstruction.[11,12] Evidence suggests that the ALL may be attached to the avulsed fragment of bone from the lateral tibial plateau seen in the setting of a Segond fracture (also known as lateral capsular sign), a radiographic finding commonly associated with ACL injury.[13,14]

The purpose of this systematic review was to describe the quality of literature on the ALL from January 1, 2000, to December 3, 2016. A systematic review of literature for quality and sources on this topic has not yet been conducted. It is hypothesized that since the "rediscovery" of the ALL, the quality of ALL-focused literature has improved and the quantity of literature available has increased.

MATERIALS AND METHODS

This study was conducted according to the methods used by Ayeni and colleagues.[15] It is reported according to the Preferred Reporting Items for Systematic Reviews and Meta-Analyses (PRISMA) statement.[16]

Study Eligibility

Studies meeting the following inclusion criterion were included in this review: any publication featuring all levels of evidence in a peer-reviewed journal primarily focused on the ALL, published between January 1, 2000, and December 3, 2016. This search range was chosen to capture any literature leading up, and responding to, what some investigators consider to be the "rediscovery" of the ALL in 2012 to 2013.[1,10,14] Editorial comments, letters to the editor, instructional course lectures, studies focusing on animal anatomy, and any studies not published in English were excluded.

Identification of Studies

Three databases (MEDLINE, PubMed, and EMBASE) were independently searched for studies published between January 1, 2000, and December 3, 2016. The following search terms were used: ALL, anterior band of the lateral collateral ligament, mid-third capsular ligament, anterior oblique band, anterolateral capsule, lateral capsular ligament, and capsulo-osseous layer of the iliotibial band. **Table 1** outlines the search strategy. The articles were screened for eligibility based on their titles by 2 reviewers (P.M., E.Q.). Any disputes during the title screen were resolved by including the articles for further screening. Because of the low volume of articles remaining after the title screen, abstract and full-text screening of all studies deemed potentially relevant were combined into a single process. Any disagreements at this level were resolved by a third more senior author (N. H.).

Data Extraction

Data were extracted by 2 reviewers (P.M., E.Q.) using a piloted electronic data extraction form (Microsoft Excel, version 15.2; Microsoft Corporation, Redmond, WA). The following data were extracted from all studies during full-text review: year of publication, study design, type of study, level of evidence with explanation for categorization, number of patients, gender, mean age, age range of patients, and type of journal. Studies dealing with cadaveric specimens, biomechanical

Table 1
Search strategy

	MEDLINE	EMBASE	PubMed
Search strategy	1. Hip/or hip.mp. 2. Arthroscopy/or arthroscopy.mp. 3. 1 and 2 4. Hip arthroscopy.mp. 5. Femoroacetabular impingement.mp. or Femoroacetabular impingement/ 6. Labrum 7. Hip/or hip.mp. 8. 6 and 7 9. 3 or 4 or 5 or 8 10. Age 11. Old 12. Elderly 13. Osteoarthritis.mp. or osteoarthritis/ 14. Years.mp. 15. 10 or 11 or 12 or 13 or 14 16. 9 and 15 17. Limit 16 to (English language and humans)	1. Hip/or hip.mp. 2. Arthroscopy/or arthroscopy.mp. 3. 1 and 2 4. Hip arthroscopy.mp. 5. Femoroacetabular impingement.mp. or Femoroacetabular impingement/ 6. Labrum 7. Hip/or hip.mp. 8. 6 and 7 9. 3 or 4 or 5 or 8 10. Age 11. Old 12. Elderly 13. Osteoarthritis.mp. or osteoarthritis/ 14. Years.mp. 15. 10 or 11 or 12 or 13 or 14 16. 9 and 15 Limit 16 to (English language and humans)	(((Hip) AND (Arthroscopy)) OR (hip arthroscopy) OR (femoroacetabular impingement) OR ((labrum) AND (hip))) AND age) AND ((old) OR (elderly) OR (osteoarthritis) OR (years))
Number of papers retrieved	1575	1796	657

data, and/or histologic analysis were classified as basic science study type. Decisions regarding ambiguous journal types were made based on the mission statement provided by the journal. The level of evidence was evaluated based on the definitions set out by the Oxford Center for Evidence-based Medicine (OCEBM) guidelines.[17] The quality of cadaveric studies was further evaluated using the Quality Appraisal for Cadaveric Studies (QUACS) 13-point scale.[18] Non–randomized controlled studies were evaluated by the Methodological Index for Non-randomized Studies (MINORS) instrument 16-point scale for noncomparative and 24-point scale for comparative nonrandomized surgical studies.[19]

Data Analysis

Interobserver agreement for reviewers' assessments of study eligibility was calculated with the Cohen kappa (k) coefficient.[20] On the basis of the recommendations of Landis and Koch,[20] a k of 0 to 0.2 represents slight agreement; 0.21 to 0.40, fair agreement; 0.41 to 0.60, moderate agreement; and 0.61 to 0.80, substantial agreement. A value greater than 0.80 is considered to indicate almost perfect agreement. Descriptive statistics were used to summarize the data. All analyses were performed using Microsoft Excel (version 15.2; Microsoft Corporation).

RESULTS
Identification of Studies

The electronic search from 3 databases returned 3441 results, 1567 of which were removed as duplicates. This left 1874 studies eligible for title review. Exclusion criteria were applied to these articles, resulting in the removal of 1665 articles. The remaining 209 studies underwent combined abstract and full-text review whereby an additional

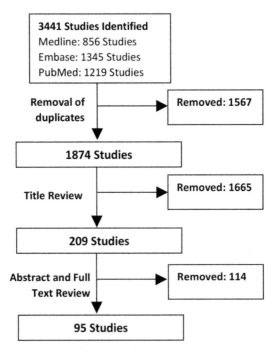

Fig. 1. Flowchart of article identification and exclusion.

114 articles were removed. A total of 95 studies were eligible for inclusion in this systematic review (**Fig. 1**). A list of included studies can be found in **Table 2**. The overall agreement between reviewers (P.M., E.Q.) was substantial with a kappa of 0.86 (95% confidence interval [CI] 0.82–0.90) at title screen and 0.96 (95% CI 0.90–1.02) during the combined abstract and full-text review.

Characteristics of Included Studies

The total number of subjects included in this systematic review was 2438; 1179 cadaveric specimens and 1259 patients. The median number of specimens used in cadaveric studies patients was 13 (interquartile range [IQR] 10.0–33.5). The median number of subjects in patient studies was 41 (IQR 12.25–77.25). The overall median sample size for all subject types was 15 (IQR 10.0–42.5). Sex distribution was not equal among the included studies, resulting in data from a total of 1048 male individuals (534 cadavers, 514 patients) and 599 female individuals (327 cadavers, 272 patients). The weighted mean age of participants was 49.8 years (cadaveric 40.8 years, patient 20.5 years) and the range of patient ages across all included articles was 3 months to 103 years. Articles not reporting relevant patient characteristics were excluded from the respective demographics calculations.

Literature and Source Trends

There were no articles with a primary focus on the ALL published between January 1, 2000, and December 31, 2011. From January 1, 2012, onward, the amount of ALL-focused literature produced each year has increased substantially (**Fig. 2**). Only 1 ALL-focused article was identified in 2012, whereas 45 articles were identified for the period of January 1, 2016, to December 3, 2016. The research published during the latter period contributed to 47.4% of all literature on the ALL. No decrease in publication volume was noted year to year.

All articles identified in this review were level 4 or 5 quality evidence according to OCEBM definitions .[17] There were 19 level 4 studies (20.0%) and 76 level 5 studies (80.0%). The number of level 5 articles has grown at a greater rate than level 4 articles (see **Fig. 2**). No randomized controlled studies involving the ALL were identified. The mean score of the 53 included cadaveric studies as assessed using the 13-point QUACS scale was 9.63 (SD 2.77). The mean MINORS scores for the 21 noncomparative and 10 comparative non–randomized controlled studies were 4.4 (SD 2.9) and 7.5 (SD 2.3), respectively. QUACS and MINORS scoring can be found in **Table 2** for applicable studies.

The study design of many of the included articles was biomechanical/cadaveric (60.0%) studies, followed by radiographic studies (18.9%). A similar number of clinical (11.6%) and review (9.5%) articles were identified (**Fig. 3**). Among the included review articles, 7 were narrative reviews and 2 were systematic reviews describing structure, function, biomechanics, and histology. There was a notable increase in the number of biomechanical/cadaveric-based articles published in 2016. The literature produced in this period comprised 50.8% of studies within the biomechanical/cadaveric category and 30.5% of all studies focusing on the ALL.

Because a significant portion of the articles were biomechanical/cadaveric studies aiming to characterize the ALL, the study type was basic science in most cases (71.5%) (**Fig. 4**). The most common study types among the remaining articles were therapeutic (13.7%), followed by diagnostic (9.5%), then prevalence (3.2%) and prognostic (1.1%). There was 1 article focused on both diagnostic and therapeutic findings.

Articles with a primary focus on the ALL were published predominantly in orthopedic journals (54.7%). Other journal types in which articles featuring the ALL frequently

Table 2
Included studies and data extracted

Author, Citation Number	Study Design	Level of Evidence (OCEBM)	Type of Study	No. Patients/Study	Female, %	Male, %	Age of Participant, y, Mean (Range)	Type of Journal (Specialty)	QUACS Score	MINORS Score
Rahnemai-Azar et al,[27] 2016	Biomechanical/Cadaveric	5	Not applicable	9	11.1	88.9	57	Sport medicine	10	N/A
Nitri et al,[28] 2016	Biomechanical/Cadaveric	5	Therapeutic	10	0	100	49.3 (41–64)	Sport medicine	11	N/A
Rasmussen et al,[29] 2016	Biomechanical/Cadaveric	5	Therapeutic	10	0	100	49.3 (41–64)	Sport medicine	10	N/A
Helito et al,[30] 2016	Biomechanical/Cadaveric	5	Therapeutic	48	10.4	89.6		Orthopedic	11	N/A
Caterine et al,[31] 2015	Biomechanical/Cadaveric	5	Not applicable	16	43.8	81.3	70 (51–94)	Orthopedic	12	N/A
Lutz et al,[32] 2015	Biomechanical/Cadaveric	5	Not applicable	9	55.6	44.4	77.7 (63–86)	Orthopedic	11	N/A
Zens et al,[33] 2015	Biomechanical/Cadaveric	5	Not applicable	6	33.3	66.7	86.7	Sport medicine	11	N/A
Spencer et al,[3] 2015	Biomechanical/Cadaveric	5	Not applicable	12	33.3	66.7	74	Sport medicine	11	N/A
Kennedy et al,[34] 2015	Biomechanical/Cadaveric	5	Not applicable	15	0	100	58.2 (39–69)	Sport medicine	10	N/A
Parsons et al,[35] 2015	Biomechanical/Cadaveric	5	Not applicable	11			76.3 (36–92)	Sport medicine	11	N/A
Claes et al,[14] 2014	Biomechanical/Cadaveric	5	Not applicable	56	33.9	66.1	59	Orthopedic	11	N/A
Helito et al,[36] 2014	Biomechanical/Cadaveric	5	Not applicable	10	0	100	62.8 (49–77)	Sport medicine	12	N/A

Study	Type		Design					Specialty		
Dodds et al,[37] 2014	Biomechanical/ Cadaveric	5	Not applicable	40				Orthopedic	10	N/A
Claes et al,[38] 2013	Biomechanical/ Cadaveric	5	Not applicable	41	46.3	53.7	79 (61–93)	Musculoskeletal	10	N/A
Vincent et al,[39] 2012	Biomechanical/ Cadaveric	5	Not applicable	40	20	5	85.3	Orthopedic	N/A	N/A
Imbert et al,[40] 2016	Biomechanical/ Cadaveric	5	Not applicable	12	66.7	33.3	76.4 (64.5–87.2)	Orthopedic	11	N/A
Wytrykowski et al,[41] 2016	Biomechanical/ Cadaveric	5	Not applicable	13	53.8	46.2	54 (37–70)	Orthopedic	12	N/A
Kosy et al,[42] 2016	Biomechanical/ Cadaveric	5	Not applicable	11	81.8	18.2	78.2 (71–88)	Orthopedic	10	N/A
Shea et al,[43] 2017	Biomechanical/ Cadaveric	5	Not applicable	14	14.3	85.7	8.6 (7–11)	Orthopedic	13	N/A
Watanabe et al,[44] 2016	Biomechanical/ Cadaveric	5	Prevalence	54	55.6	44.4	85.6 (70–103)	Orthopedic	9	N/A
Coquart et al,[45] 2016	Biomechanical/ Cadaveric	5	Diagnostic	71	45.1	40.8	48 (15–83)	Musculoskeletal	11	N/A
Kennedy et al,[46] 2015	Biomechanical/ Cadaveric	5	Not applicable	15				Orthopedic	3	N/A
Helito et al,[47] 2013	Biomechanical/ Cadaveric	5	Not applicable	20	20	80	61.5 (37–67)	Orthopedic	10	N/A
Thein et al,[48] 2016	Biomechanical/ Cadaveric	5	Not applicable	12	33.3	66.7	43 (20–64)	Orthopedic	11	N/A
Parker and Smith,[49] 2016	Biomechanical/ Cadaveric	5	Not applicable	53	50.9	49.1		Basic science	3	N/A
Hinkley et al,[50] 2016	Biomechanical/ Cadaveric	5	Prevalence	41				Basic science	4	N/A

(continued on next page)

Table 2
(continued)

Author, Citation Number	Study Design	Level of Evidence (OCEBM)	Type of Study	No. Patients/ Study	Female, %	Male, %	Age of Participant, y, Mean (Range)	Type of Journal (Specialty)	QUACS Score	MINORS Score
Shea et al,[51] 2016	Biomechanical/ Cadaveric	5	Not applicable	8	62.5	37.5	3.44 (0.25–10)	Orthopedic	8	N/A
Heckmann et al,[52] 2016	Biomechanical/ Cadaveric	5	Not applicable	12			68.4	Orthopedic	12	N/A
Macchi et al,[53] 2016	Biomechanical/ Cadaveric	5	Not applicable	60	40	60	59.9	Radiology	9	N/A
Daggett et al,[54] 2016	Biomechanical/ Cadaveric	5	Not applicable					Orthopedic	5	N/A
Runer et al,[55] 2016	Biomechanical/ Cadaveric	5	Not applicable	50	56	44	78.1 (61–94)	Musculoskeletal	11	N/A
Helito et al,[56] 2016	Biomechanical/ Cadaveric	5	Not applicable	33	0	100	60.1	Radiology	11	N/A
Helito et al,[57] 2015	Biomechanical/ Cadaveric	5	Not applicable	13	0	100	66 (49–82)	Orthopedic	12	N/A
Zens et al,[58] 2015	Biomechanical/ Cadaveric	5	Not applicable	4	25	75	85.6	Orthopedic	11	N/A
Helito et al,[59] 2014	Biomechanical/ Cadaveric	5	Not applicable	10	20	80		Orthopedic	10	N/A
Alimohammadi,[60] 2014	Biomechanical/ Cadaveric	5	Not applicable	34	41.2	58.8		Basic science	2	N/A
Caterine et al,[61] 2014	Biomechanical/ Cadaveric	5	Not applicable	7				Basic science	2	N/A
Claes et al,[62] 2013	Biomechanical/ Cadaveric	5	Not applicable	41				Orthopedic	4	N/A

			Prevalence					Medicine	9	N/A
Potu et al,[63] 2016	Biomechanical/Cadaveric	5		24				Medicine	9	N/A
Bonanzinga et al,[64] 2016	Biomechanical/Cadaveric	5	Not applicable	5			79	Orthopedic	11	N/A
Helito et al,[65] 2017	Biomechanical/Cadaveric	5	Not applicable	20	50	50	0.549 (0.48–0.71)	Sport medicine	12	N/A
Schon et al,[66] 2016	Biomechanical/Cadaveric	5	Therapeutic	10	0	100	55.9 (46–64)	Sport medicine	12	N/A
Capo et al,[67] 2016	Biomechanical/Cadaveric	5	Not applicable	10				Orthopedic	10	N/A
Van de Velde et al,[68] 2016	Biomechanical/Cadaveric	5	Not applicable	10	40	60		Sport medicine	N/A	N/A
Katakura et al,[69] 2016	Biomechanical/Cadaveric	5	Therapeutic	6	33.3	66.7		Orthopedic	12	N/A
Helito et al,[70] 2016	Biomechanical/Cadaveric	5	Not applicable	14	0	100	62.6 (49–77)	Medicine	11	N/A
Sonnery-Cottet et al,[71] 2016	Biomechanical/Cadaveric	5	Not applicable	12	66.7	33.3	76.4 (65.4–87.2)	Sport medicine	10	N/A
Daggett et al,[72] 2016	Biomechanical/Cadaveric	5	Not applicable	52	42.3	57.7		Orthopedic	11	N/A
Saiegh et al,[73] 2015	Biomechanical/Cadaveric	5	Not applicable	3	33.3	66.7	42	Orthopedic	10	N/A
Tavlo et al,[74] 2016	Biomechanical/Cadaveric	5	Not applicable	18	22.2	77.8	77.8	Sport medicine	11	N/A
Dombrowski et al,[75] 2016	Biomechanical/Cadaveric	5	Not applicable	10	40	60	55.9 (19–68)	Orthopedic	9	N/A
Stijak et al,[76] 2016	Biomechanical/Cadaveric	5	Not applicable	14	57.1	42.9	78	Orthopedic	10	N/A

(continued on next page)

Table 2
(continued)

Author, Citation Number	Study Design	Level of Evidence (OCEBM)	Type of Study	No. Patients/Study	Female, %	Male, %	Age of Participant, y, Mean (Range)	Type of Journal (Specialty)	QUACS Score	MINORS Score
Sonnery-Cottet et al,[77] 2014	Biomechanical/Cadaveric	5	Diagnostic					Orthopedic	5	N/A
Kittl et al,[78] 2016	Biomechanical/Cadaveric	5	Not applicable	16	50	50	69 (52–93)	Sport medicine	11	N/A
Rezansoff et al,[79] 2015	Biomechanical/Cadaveric	5	Not applicable	13	38.5	61.5	70.8	Orthopedic	12	N/A
Cavaignac et al,[80] 2016	Biomechanical/Cadaveric	5	Not applicable	18	66.7	33.3	84 (77–90)	Orthopedic	11	N/A
Zens et al,[81] 2014	Biomechanical/Cadaveric	5	Not applicable		100	0	82 (73–87)	Prevalence	8	N/A
Sonnery-Cottet et al,[12] 2015	Clinical	4	Therapeutic	92	26.1	73.9	24	Sport medicine	N/A	13
Ferretti et al,[82] 2017	Clinical	4	Therapeutic	60	31.7	68.3	24 (18–35)	Orthopedic	N/A	7
Davis et al,[83] 2015	Clinical	5	More than one	2	0	100	35.3 (29–42)	Radiology	N/A	6
Smith et al,[84] 2015	Clinical	5	Therapeutic					Orthopedic	N/A	1
Cianca et al,[85] 2014	Clinical	5	Diagnostic	1	0	100	52	Medicine	N/A	5
Wagih et al,[86] 2016	Clinical	5	Therapeutic					Orthopedic	N/A	2

Study	Type		Purpose	n				Specialty		
Chahla et al,[11] 2016	Clinical	5	Therapeutic					Orthopedic	N/A	2
Figueroa et al,[87] 2016	Clinical	5	Therapeutic					Orthopedic	N/A	2
Sonnery-Cottet et al,[88] 2016	Clinical	5	Therapeutic					Orthopedic	N/A	2
Zein,[89] 2015	Clinical	5	Not applicable					Orthopedic	N/A	2
Ferreira et al,[90] 2016	Clinical	5	Therapeutic	15	20	80		Orthopedic	N/A	2
Hartigan et al,[91] 2016	Radiology	4	Diagnostic	72				Orthopedic	N/A	8
Kosy et al,[92] 2015	Radiology	4	Diagnostic	98	35.7	64.3	45.3 (16–85)	Radiology	N/A	3
Klontzas et al,[93] 2016	Radiology	4	Diagnostic	43	27.9	51.2	28.7	Radiology	N/A	7
Taneja et al,[94] 2015	Radiology	4	Not applicable	60	46.7	53.3	40 (11–75)	Radiology	N/A	9
Porrino et al,[95] 2015	Radiology	4	Not applicable	73	52.1	47.9		Radiology	N/A	6
Helito et al,[96] 2014	Radiology	4	Diagnostic	39	33.3	66.7		Radiology	N/A	11
Claes et al,[97] 2014	Radiology	4	Diagnostic	206				Orthopedic	N/A	3

(continued on next page)

Table 2
(continued)

Author, Citation Number	Study Design	Level of Evidence (OCEBM)	Type of Study	No. Patients/Study	Female, %	Male, %	Age of Participant, y, Mean (Range)	Type of Journal (Specialty)	QUACS Score	MINORS Score
Kernkamp et al,[98] 2017	Radiology	4	Not applicable	18	33.3	66.7	35.4	Orthopedic	N/A	7
Flores et al,[99] 2016	Radiology	4	Not applicable	146				Radiology	N/A	3
Van Dyck et al,[100] 2016	Radiology	4	Diagnostic	90	26.7	73.3	32 (17–59)	Radiology	N/A	7
Hurley et al,[101] 2015	Radiology	4	Prognostic	10				Medicine	N/A	5
Oshima et al,[102] 2016	Radiology	4	Not applicable	9	0	100	30.3 (28–37)	Musculoskeletal	N/A	11
Wodicka et al,[103] 2014	Radiology	4	Not applicable	50				Orthopedic	N/A	2
Helito et al,[104] 2017	Radiology	4	Not applicable	101	21.8	78.2	33.5	Orthopedic	N/A	7
Yokosawa et al,[105] 2016	Radiology	4	Not applicable	27	14.8	85.2	37	Radiology	N/A	6
Helito et al,[106] 2015	Radiology	4	Not applicable	33	78.8	21.2	32.5 (21–49)	Orthopedic	N/A	4

Study										
De Maeseneer et al,[107] 2015	Radiology	4	Not applicable	13	46.2	53.8	36 (17–52)	Radiology	N/A	5
Mahajer,[108] 2014	Radiology	5	Not applicable	1	0	100	31 (31–31)	Physiotherapy	N/A	6
Van der Watt et al,[1] 2015	Review	5	Not applicable					Orthopedic	N/A	N/A
Pomajzl et al,[9]	Review	5	Not applicable					Orthopedic	N/A	N/A
Kosy et al,[109]	Review	5	Not applicable					Orthopedic	N/A	N/A
Feucht et al,[110] 2016	Review	5	Not applicable					Orthopedic	N/A	N/A
Van Dyck et al,[111] 2016	Review	5	Not applicable					Radiology	N/A	N/A
Roessler et al,[112] 2016	Review	5	Not applicable					Orthopedic	N/A	N/A
Bonasia et al,[113] 2015	Review	5	Not applicable					Orthopedic	N/A	N/A
Cavaignac et al,[114] 2016	Review	5	Not applicable					Sport medicine	N/A	N/A
Guenther et al,[115] 2015	Review	5	Not applicable					Orthopedic	N/A	N/A

Red indicates unreported data.

Abbreviations: MINORS, Methodological Index for Non-randomized Studies; N/A, not available; OCEBM, Oxford Center for Evidence-based Medicine; QUACS, Quality Appraisal for Cadaveric Studies.

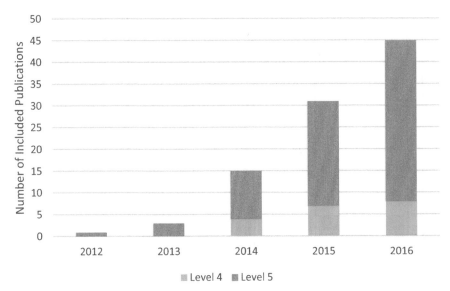

Fig. 2. Number of publications with a focus on the ALL per year.

appeared included sports medicine (16.8%), radiology (13.7%), medicine (4.2%), basic science (4.2%), musculoskeletal (4.2%), physiotherapy (1.0%), and computer technology (1.0%).

DISCUSSION
Key Findings

This systematic review found an increased rate in the number of ALL-focused publications since 2012. To our knowledge, this is the first systematic review to examine the subject matter and quality of the ALL literature. Our results confirmed that there were no articles focusing primarily on the ALL published between 2000 and 2012. The number of new articles published each year has increased substantially, with 45 articles published in 2016 compared with a single publication in 2012. Nonetheless, given the total of 95 low-level studies identified in this review, the overall quantity of literature regarding the ALL remains small. Although lacking in volume, most currently available

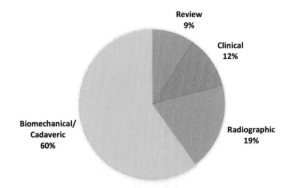

Fig. 3. Proportion of included studies categorized by study design.

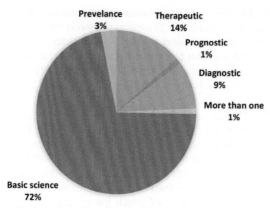

Fig. 4. Proportion of included articles classified by study type.

literature regarding the ALL supports its existence as an independent anterolateral capsular structure of the knee.

The median sample size of ALL publications using both cadaveric and live subjects included in this review was 15 (IQR 10.0–42.5). Studies of small sample size are at risk of bias, as they are likely underpowered.[21,22] These articles are helpful in generating hypotheses, but cannot be used reliably to make general conclusions about the ALL given their inherent limitations.[23]

The overall level of evidence among the included studies was low, as no studies with level 1 to 3 evidence were identified. Although level 5 evidence constituted most of the literature on the ALL, the volume of level 4 studies has been increasing in recent years. Despite falling into the level 5 evidence category, the cadaveric studies scored a mean of 74.1% on the QUACS scale, indicating good methodological quality. Conversely, the vast majority of noncomparative and comparative non–randomized controlled studies pertaining to the ALL scored poorly on the MINORS scale, with means of 4.4 (SD 2.9) and 7.5 (SD 2.3), respectively. This demonstrates a general low methodological quality of noncadaveric literature on the ALL. A single noncomparative study published in 2015 was shown to be of good methodologic quality, with a MINORS score of 13, indicating that robust research into the ALL is feasible albeit currently lacking.[12] The low methodologic quality of non–randomized controlled studies at present is thought to be in part due to strict exclusion criteria applied by nearly half of the reviewed literature, whereby knees with current or prior injuries were excluded from analysis. Although this substantially limits sample size and the resulting methodologic robustness, it is an understandable criterion, because the fundamental purpose of these articles is to establish the feasibility of diagnostic imaging and biomechanical roles of the ALL.

It was noted that 60% of the identified articles were biomechanical/cadaveric in nature, suggesting that both the structure and function of the ALL is not yet fully understood. Clinical and radiographic studies comprise 30.5% of the included literature. Although these study designs have demonstrated growth, they have been outpaced by biomechanical/cadaveric literature, particularly in 2016. This systematic review identifies a need for more clinical and radiographic studies to expand knowledge regarding the role of the ALL in ligamentous knee injury.

There are few clinical studies addressing the ALL. As a result of its recent "rediscovery," clinically oriented high level-of-evidence studies on this structure are lacking. Data on the frequency of ALL reconstruction or lateral extra-articular tenodesis could not be identified, and an apparent lack of clear indications for either procedure may be making the transition from cadaveric to clinical research difficult.[24] Recent entries for randomized controlled trials involving combined ACL reconstruction and ALL reconstruction or lateral extra-articular tenodesis can be found in a clinical trials database. These studies will analyze data on rotational knee stability and patient-reported outcome measures using the Knee Number-Entity Evaluation Score.[25,26]

Strengths and Limitations

This systematic review used broad search terms in attempt to capture all studies related to the ALL. Duplicate reviewer screening and inclusion for full-text review in cases of disagreement ensured thorough evaluation of potentially relevant literature. High interrater agreement suggests well-defined, a priori-designed inclusion criteria.

Given the current lack of standardized terminology for the ALL, there may have been additional nomenclature for the ALL of which the researchers were not aware. No other terms were identified during literature analysis for this systematic review, thus the possibility that our search was not exhaustive is small. Our review excluded publications that were not published in the English language, thereby creating a language and publication bias. Nevertheless, a total of 4 papers for which English translations existed were included in our review.

SUMMARY

Although there has been a notable increase in the number of ALL-focused studies published since 2012, the total volume of literature on this topic is limited and composed of low-quality evidence. The generally small sample size noted among the included studies increases the risk of bias. Biomechanical/cadaveric-based studies comprise a large proportion of publications on the ALL. There are few studies pertaining to the diagnosis, therapy, prevalence, or prognosis of injury to the ALL. The volume, quality, and diversity of research on the ALL is likely to increase, as the ground work for future clinical studies has been well established through the existing basic science research available on the ALL. Future large clinical studies will help further define not only the function of the ALL but also the role of ALL reconstruction or lateral extra-articular tenodesis in the setting concomitant ACL reconstruction.

REFERENCES

1. Van der Watt L, Khan M, Rothrauff BB, et al. The structure and function of the anterolateral ligament of the knee: a systematic review. Arthroscopy 2015; 31(3):569–82.e3.
2. Segond P. Recherches cliniques et expérimentales sur les épanchements sanguins du genou par entorse. Paris: Aux bureaux du Progrès médical 1879;7: 297–334.
3. Spencer L, Burkhart TA, Tran MN, et al. Biomechanical analysis of simulated clinical testing and reconstruction of the anterolateral ligament of the knee. Am J Sports Med 2015;43(9):2189–97.
4. Terry GC, Hughston JC, Norwood LA. The anatomy of the iliopatellar band and iliotibial tract. Am J Sports Med 1986;14(1):39–45.
5. LaPrade RF, Gilbert TJ, Bollom TS, et al. The magnetic resonance imaging appearance of individual structures of the posterolateral knee. A prospective study of normal knees and knees with surgically verified grade III injuries. Am J Sports Med 2000;28(2):191–9.

6. Irvine GB, Dias JJ, Finlay DB. Segond fractures of the lateral tibial condyle: brief report. J Bone Joint Surg Br 1987;69(4):613–4.
7. Campos JC, Chung CB, Lektrakul N, et al. Pathogenesis of the Segond fracture: anatomic and MR imaging evidence of an iliotibial tract or anterior oblique band avulsion. Radiology 2001;219(2):381–6.
8. Vieira EL, Vieira EA, Da Silva RT, et al. An anatomic study of the iliotibial tract. Arthroscopy 2007;23(3):269–74.
9. Pomajzl R, Maerz T, Shams C, et al. A review of the anterolateral ligament of the knee: current knowledge regarding its incidence, anatomy, biomechanics, and surgical dissection. Arthroscopy 2015;31(3):583–91.
10. Parsons EM, Gee AO, Spiekerman C, et al. The biomechanical function of the anterolateral ligament of the knee. Am J Sports Med 2015;43(3):669–74.
11. Chahla J, Menge TJ, Mitchell JJ, et al. Anterolateral ligament reconstruction technique: an anatomic-based approach. Arthrosc Tech 2016;5(3):e453–7.
12. Sonnery-Cottet B, Thaunat M, Freychet B, et al. Outcome of a combined anterior cruciate ligament and anterolateral ligament reconstruction technique with a minimum 2-year follow-up. Am J Sports Med 2015;43(7):1598–605.
13. Woods GW, Stanley RF, Tullos HS. Lateral capsular sign: x-ray clue to a significant knee instability. Am J Sports Med 1979;7(1):27–33.
14. Claes S, Luyckx T, Vereecke E, et al. The Segond fracture: a bony injury of the anterolateral ligament of the knee. Arthroscopy 2014;30(11):1475–82.
15. Ayeni OR, Chan K, Al-asiri J, et al. Sources and quality of literature addressing femoroacetabular impingement. Knee Surg Sports Traumatol Arthrosc 2013; 21(2):415–9.
16. Moher D, Liberati A, Tetzlaff J, et al. Preferred reporting items for systematic reviews and meta-analyses: the PRISMA statement. J Clin Epidemiol 2009;62: 1006–12.
17. Oxford Centre for Evidence-based Medicine - Levels of Evidence (March 2009) - CEBM. CEBM. 2017. Available at: http://www.cebm.net/oxford-centre-evidence-based-medicine-levels-evidence-march-2009/. Accessed January 18, 2017.
18. Wilke J, Krause F, Niederer D, et al. Appraising the methodological quality of cadaveric studies: validation of the QUACS scale. J Anat 2015;226(5):440–6.
19. Slim K, Nini E, Forestier D, et al. Methological index for non-randomized studies (MINORS): development and validation of a new instrument. ANZ J Surg 2003; 73(9):712–6.
20. Landis JR, Koch GG. The measurement of observer agreement for categorical data. Biometrics 1977;33(1):159–74.
21. Guyatt GH, Oxman AD, Vist G, et al. GRADE guidelines: 4. Rating the quality of evidence–study limitations (risk of bias). J Clin Epidemiol 2011;64(4):407–15.
22. Bhandari M, Tornetta P, Rampersad SA, et al. (Sample) size matters! An examination of sample size from the SPRINT trial study to prospectively evaluate reamed intramedullary nails in patients with tibial fractures. J Orthop Trauma 2013;27(4):183–8.
23. Chaudhry H, Mundi R, Singh I, et al. How good is the orthopaedic literature? Indian J Orthop 2008;42(2):144–9.
24. Vundelinckx B, Herman B, Getgood A, et al. Surgical indications and technique for anterior cruciate ligament reconstruction combined with lateral extra-articular tenodesis or anterolateral ligament reconstruction. Clin Sports Med 2017;36(1): 135–53.
25. Komzak M. Stability of the knee joint after anterior cruciate ligament and anterolateral ligament reconstruction. Full Text View. ClinicalTrials.gov.

Clinicaltrialsgov. 2017. Available at: https://clinicaltrials.gov/ct2/show/NCT02993679?term=Anterolateral+Ligament&rank=1. Accessed January 18, 2017.

26. Martin L. Reconstruction of the anterolateral ligament (ALL) with revision anterior cruciate ligament (ACL) surgery. Full Text View. ClinicalTrials.gov. Clinicaltrialsgov. 2017. Available at: https://clinicaltrials.gov/ct2/show/NCT02680821?term=Anterolateral+Ligament&rank=2. Accessed January 18, 2017.

27. Rahnemai-azar AA, Miller RM, Guenther D, et al. Structural properties of the anterolateral capsule and iliotibial band of the knee. Am J Sports Med 2016;44(4): 892–7.

28. Nitri M, Rasmussen MT, Williams BT, et al. An in vitro robotic assessment of the anterolateral ligament, part 2: anterolateral ligament reconstruction combined with anterior cruciate ligament reconstruction. Am J Sports Med 2016;44(3): 593–601.

29. Rasmussen MT, Nitri M, Williams BT, et al. An in vitro robotic assessment of the anterolateral ligament, part 1: secondary role of the anterolateral ligament in the setting of an anterior cruciate ligament injury. Am J Sports Med 2016;44(3): 585–92.

30. Helito CP, Bonadio MB, Gobbi RG, et al. Is it safe to reconstruct the knee anterolateral ligament with a femoral tunnel? Frequency of lateral collateral ligament and popliteus tendon injury. Int Orthop 2016;40(4):821–5.

31. Caterine S, Litchfield R, Johnson M, et al. A cadaveric study of the anterolateral ligament: re-introducing the lateral capsular ligament. Knee Surg Sports Traumatol Arthrosc 2015;23(11):3186–95.

32. Lutz C, Sonnery-cottet B, Niglis L, et al. Behavior of the anterolateral structures of the knee during internal rotation. Orthop Traumatol Surg Res 2015;101(5): 523–8.

33. Zens M, Niemeyer P, Ruhhammer J, et al. Length changes of the anterolateral ligament during passive knee motion: a human cadaveric study. Am J Sports Med 2015;43(10):2545–52.

34. Kennedy MI, Claes S, Fuso FA, et al. The anterolateral ligament: an anatomic, radiographic, and biomechanical analysis. Am J Sports Med 2015;43(7): 1606–15.

35. Parsons EM, Gee AO, Spiekerman C, et al. The biomechanical function of the anterolateral ligament of the knee: response. Am J Sports Med 2015;43(8): NP22.

36. Helito CP, Demange MK, Bonadio MB, et al. Radiographic landmarks for locating the femoral origin and tibial insertion of the knee anterolateral ligament. Am J Sports Med 2014;42(10):2356–62.

37. Dodds AL, Halewood C, Gupte CM, et al. The anterolateral ligament: anatomy, length changes and association with the Segond fracture. Bone Joint J 2014; 96-B(3):325–31.

38. Claes S, Vereecke E, Maes M, et al. Anatomy of the anterolateral ligament of the knee. J Anat 2013;223(4):321–8.

39. Vincent JP, Magnussen RA, Gezmez F, et al. The anterolateral ligament of the human knee: an anatomic and histologic study. Knee Surg Sports Traumatol Arthrosc 2012;20(1):147–52.

40. Imbert P, Lutz C, Daggett M, et al. Isometric characteristics of the anterolateral ligament of the knee: a cadaveric navigation study. Arthroscopy 2016;32(10): 2017–24.

41. Wytrykowski K, Swider P, Reina N, et al. Cadaveric study comparing the biomechanical properties of grafts used for knee anterolateral ligament reconstruction. Arthroscopy 2016;32(11):2288–94.
42. Kosy JD, Soni A, Venkatesh R, et al. The anterolateral ligament of the knee: unwrapping the enigma. Anatomical study and comparison to previous reports. J Orthop Traumatol 2016;17(4):303–8.
43. Shea KG, Milewski MD, Cannamela PC, et al. Anterolateral ligament of the knee shows variable anatomy in pediatric specimens. Clin Orthop Relat Res 2016; 475(6):1583–91.
44. Watanabe J, Suzuki D, Mizoguchi S, et al. The anterolateral ligament in a Japanese population: study on prevalence and morphology. J Orthop Sci 2016;21(5): 647–51.
45. Coquart B, Le corroller T, Laurent PE, et al. Anterolateral ligament of the knee: myth or reality? Surg Radiol Anat 2016;38(8):955–62.
46. Kennedy MI, Claes S, Fuso F, et al. The anterolateral ligament (ALL): a comprehensive study encompassing anatomic and radiographic landmarks and native structural properties. Orthop J Sports Med 2015;3(7Suppl 2). 2325967115S00126.
47. Helito CP, Demange MK, Bonadio MB, et al. Anatomy and histology of the knee anterolateral ligament. Orthop J Sports Med 2013;1(7). 2325967113513546.
48. Thein R, Boorman-padgett J, Stone K, et al. Biomechanical assessment of the anterolateral ligament of the knee: a secondary restraint in simulated tests of the pivot shift and of anterior stability. J Bone Joint Surg Am 2016;98(11): 937–43.
49. Parker MF, Smith HF. An expansion of the anatomy of the anterolateral ligament of the knee: morphological variation and an alternate dissection approach. FASEB J 2016;30(1 Suppl):1043.3.
50. Hinkley J, Lampert P, Canby C. Prevalence of the anterolateral ligament. FASEB J 2016;30(1 Suppl):1046.13.
51. Shea KG, Polousky JD, Jacobs JC, et al. The anterolateral ligament of the knee: an inconsistent finding in pediatric cadaveric specimens. J Pediatr Orthop 2016;36(5):e51–4.
52. Heckmann N, Sivasundaram L, Villacis D, et al. Radiographic landmarks for identifying the anterolateral ligament of the knee. Arthroscopy 2016;32(5): 844–8.
53. Macchi V, Porzionato A, Morra A, et al. The anterolateral ligament of the knee: a radiologic and histotopographic study. Surg Radiol Anat 2016;38(3):341–8.
54. Daggett M, Busch K, Sonnery-cottet B. Surgical dissection of the anterolateral ligament. Arthrosc Tech 2016;5(1):e185–8.
55. Runer A, Birkmaier S, Pamminger M, et al. The anterolateral ligament of the knee: a dissection study. Knee 2016;23(1):8–12.
56. Helito CP, Bonadio MB, Soares TQ, et al. The meniscal insertion of the knee anterolateral ligament. Surg Radiol Anat 2016;38(2):223–8.
57. Helito CP, Helito PV, Bonadio MB, et al. Correlation of magnetic resonance imaging with knee anterolateral ligament anatomy: a cadaveric study. Orthop J Sports Med 2015;3(12). 2325967115621024.
58. Zens M, Feucht MJ, Ruhhammer J, et al. Mechanical tensile properties of the anterolateral ligament. J Exp Orthop 2015;2(1):7.
59. Helito CP, Helito PV, Bonadio MB, et al. Evaluation of the length and isometric pattern of the anterolateral ligament with serial computer tomography. Orthop J Sports Med 2014;2(12). 2325967114562205.

60. Alimohammadi M. Incidence and structural variety of the anterior lateral ligament of the knee joint (LB12). FASEB J 2014;28(1 Suppl):LB12.

61. Caterine S, Litchfield R, Johnson M, et al. Structural characterization of the anterolateral capsule of the knee—a gross anatomic, histological, and magnetic resonance imaging study of the anterolateral ligament (914.6). FASEB J 2014; 28(1 Suppl):914.6.

62. Claes S, Vereecke E, Luyckx T, et al. The Segond fracture: just an x-ray clue for a ruptured anterior cruciate ligament? Arthroscopy 2013;29(10):e86.

63. Potu BK, Salem AH, Abu-hijleh MF. Morphology of anterolateral ligament of the knee: a cadaveric observation with clinical insight. Adv Med 2016;2016: 9182863.

64. Bonanzinga T, Signorelli C, Grassi A, et al. Kinematics of ACL and anterolateral ligament. Part I: combined lesion. Knee Surg Sports Traumatol Arthrosc 2017; 25(4):1055–61.

65. Helito CP, Do prado torres JA, Bonadio MB, et al. Anterolateral ligament of the fetal knee. Am J Sports Med 2017;45(1):91–6.

66. Schon JM, Moatshe G, Brady AW, et al. Anatomic anterolateral ligament reconstruction of the knee leads to overconstraint at any fixation angle. Am J Sports Med 2016;44(10):2540–50.

67. Capo J, Kaplan DJ, Fralinger DJ, et al. Ultrasonographic visualization and assessment of the anterolateral ligament. Knee Surg Sports Traumatol Arthrosc 2016. [Epub ahead of print].

68. Van de velde SK, Kernkamp WA, Hosseini A, et al. In vivo length changes of the anterolateral ligament and related extra-articular reconstructions. Am J Sports Med 2016;44(10):2557–62.

69. Katakura M, Koga H, Nakamura K, et al. Effects of different femoral tunnel positions on tension changes in anterolateral ligament reconstruction. Knee Surg Sports Traumatol Arthrosc 2017;25(4):1272–8.

70. Helito CP, Bonadio MB, Rozas JS, et al. Biomechanical study of strength and stiffness of the knee anterolateral ligament. BMC Musculoskelet Disord 2016; 17:193.

71. Sonnery-cottet B, Lutz C, Daggett M, et al. The involvement of the anterolateral ligament in rotational control of the knee. Am J Sports Med 2016;44(5):1209–14.

72. Daggett M, Ockuly AC, Cullen M, et al. Femoral origin of the anterolateral ligament: an anatomic analysis. Arthroscopy 2016;32(5):835–41.

73. Saiegh YA, Suero EM, Guenther D, et al. Sectioning the anterolateral ligament did not increase tibiofemoral translation or rotation in an ACL-deficient cadaveric model. Knee Surg Sports Traumatol Arthrosc 2017;25(4):1086–92.

74. Tavlo M, Eljaja S, Jensen JT, et al. The role of the anterolateral ligament in ACL insufficient and reconstructed knees on rotatory stability: a biomechanical study on human cadavers. Scand J Med Sci Sports 2016;26(8):960–6.

75. Dombrowski ME, Costello JM, Ohashi B, et al. Macroscopic anatomical, histological and magnetic resonance imaging correlation of the lateral capsule of the knee. Knee Surg Sports Traumatol Arthrosc 2016;24(9):2854–60.

76. Stijak L, Bumbaširević M, Radonjić V, et al. Anatomic description of the anterolateral ligament of the knee. Knee Surg Sports Traumatol Arthrosc 2016;24(7): 2083–8.

77. Sonnery-Cottet B, Archbold P, Rezende FC, et al. Arthroscopic identification of the anterolateral ligament of the knee. Arthrosc Tech 2014;3(3):e389–92.

78. Kittl C, El-daou H, Athwal KK, et al. The role of the anterolateral structures and the ACL in controlling laxity of the intact and ACL-deficient knee. Am J Sports Med 2016;44(2):345–54.

79. Rezansoff AJ, Caterine S, Spencer L, et al. Radiographic landmarks for surgical reconstruction of the anterolateral ligament of the knee. Knee Surg Sports Traumatol Arthrosc 2015;23(11):3196–201.

80. Cavaignac E, Wytrykowski K, Reina N, et al. Ultrasonographic identification of the anterolateral ligament of the knee. Arthroscopy 2016;32(1):120–6.

81. Zens M, Ruhhammer J, Goldschmidtboeing F, et al. A new approach to determine ligament strain using polydimethylsiloxane strain gauges: exemplary measurements of the anterolateral ligament. J Biomech Eng 2014;136(12):124504.

82. Ferretti A, Monaco E, Fabbri M, et al. Prevalence and classification of injuries of anterolateral complex in acute anterior cruciate ligament tears. Arthroscopy 2017;33(1):147–54.

83. Davis BA, Hiller LP, Imbesi SG, et al. Isolated lateral collateral ligament complex injury in rock climbing and Brazilian Jiu-jitsu. Skeletal Radiol 2015;44(8):1175–9.

84. Smith JO, Yasen SK, Lord B, et al. Combined anterolateral ligament and anatomic anterior cruciate ligament reconstruction of the knee. Knee Surg Sports Traumatol Arthrosc 2015;23(11):3151–6.

85. Cianca J, John J, Pandit S, et al. Musculoskeletal ultrasound imaging of the recently described anterolateral ligament of the knee. Am J Phys Med Rehabil 2014;93(2):186.

86. Wagih AM, Elguindy AM. Percutaneous reconstruction of the anterolateral ligament of the knee with a polyester tape. Arthrosc Tech 2016;5(4):e691–7.

87. Figuero D, Schmidt-Hebbel A, Calvo R, et al. Minimally invasive anterolateral ligament reconstruction following anterior cruciate ligament revision surgery. Technical note. Revista chilena de ortopedia y traumatologia 2016;57(2):36–41.

88. Sonnery-cottet B, Barbosa NC, Tuteja S, et al. Minimally invasive anterolateral ligament reconstruction in the setting of anterior cruciate ligament injury. Arthrosc Tech 2016;5(1):e211–5.

89. Zein AM. Step-by-step arthroscopic assessment of the anterolateral ligament of the knee using anatomic landmarks. Arthrosc Tech 2015;4(6):e825–31.

90. Ferreira Mde C, Zidan FF, Miduati FB, et al. Reconstruction of anterior cruciate ligament and anterolateral ligament using interlinked hamstrings—technical note. Rev Bras Ortop 2016;51(4):466–70.

91. Hartigan DE, Carroll KW, Kosarek FJ, et al. Visibility of anterolateral ligament tears in anterior cruciate ligament-deficient knees with standard 1.5-Tesla magnetic resonance imaging. Arthroscopy 2016;32(10):2061–5.

92. Kosy JD, Mandalia VI, Anaspure R. Characterization of the anatomy of the anterolateral ligament of the knee using magnetic resonance imaging. Skeletal Radiol 2015;44(11):1647–53.

93. Klontzas ME, Maris TG, Zibis AH, et al. Normal magnetic resonance imaging anatomy of the anterolateral knee ligament with a T2/T1-weighted 3-dimensional sequence: a feasibility study. Can Assoc Radiol J 2016;67(1):52–9.

94. Taneja AK, Miranda FC, Braga CA, et al. MRI features of the anterolateral ligament of the knee. Skeletal Radiol 2015;44(3):403–10.

95. Porrino J, Maloney E, Richardson M, et al. The anterolateral ligament of the knee: MRI appearance, association with the Segond fracture, and historical perspective. AJR Am J Roentgenol 2015;204(2):367–73.

96. Helito CP, Helito PV, Costa HP, et al. MRI evaluation of the anterolateral ligament of the knee: assessment in routine 1.5-T scans. Skeletal Radiol 2014;43(10): 1421–7.
97. Claes S, Bartholomeeusen S, Bellemans J. High prevalence of anterolateral ligament abnormalities in magnetic resonance images of anterior cruciate ligament-injured knees. Acta Orthop Belg 2014;80(1):45–9.
98. Kernkamp WA, Van de velde SK, Hosseini A, et al. in vivo anterolateral ligament length change in the healthy knee during functional activities-a combined magnetic resonance and dual fluoroscopic imaging analysis. Arthroscopy 2017; 33(1):133–9.
99. Flores DV, Smitaman E, Huang BK, et al. Segond fracture: an MR evaluation of 146 patients with emphasis on the avulsed bone fragment and what attaches to it. Skeletal Radiol 2016;45(12):1635–47.
100. Van dyck P, Clockaerts S, Vanhoenacker FM, et al. Anterolateral ligament abnormalities in patients with acute anterior cruciate ligament rupture are associated with lateral meniscal and osseous injuries. Eur Radiol 2016;26(10):3383–91.
101. Hurley R, Barry C, Bergin D, et al. A magnetic resonance imaging study and description of the anterolateral ligament of the knee. Ir J Med Sci 2015;184: S419–20.
102. Oshima T, Nakase J, Numata H, et al. Ultrasonography imaging of the anterolateral ligament using real-time virtual sonography. Knee 2016;23(2):198–202.
103. Wodicka R, Jose J, Baraga MG, et al. Evaluation of the anterolateral ligament of the knee in the setting of ACL rupture. Orthop J Sports Med 2014;2(2 Suppl). 2325967114S00042.
104. Helito CP, Helito PV, Costa HP, et al. Assessment of the anterolateral ligament of the knee by magnetic resonance imaging in acute injuries of the anterior cruciate ligament. Arthroscopy 2017;33(1):140–6.
105. Yokosawa K, Sasaki K, Muramatsu K, et al. Visualization of anterolateral ligament of the knee using 3D reconstructed variable refocus flip angle-turbo spin echo T2 weighted image. Nihon Hoshasen Gijutsu Gakkai Zasshi 2016; 72(5):416–23 [in Japanese].
106. Helito CP, Demange MK, Helito PV, et al. Evaluation of the anterolateral ligament of the knee by means of magnetic resonance examination. Rev Bras Ortop 2015;50(2):214–9.
107. De maeseneer M, Boulet C, Willekens I, et al. Segond fracture: involvement of the iliotibial band, anterolateral ligament, and anterior arm of the biceps femoris in knee trauma. Skeletal Radiol 2015;44(3):413–21.
108. Mahajer A. Poster 271 lateral geniculate artery a key anatomy landmark in sonographic evaluation of the anterolateral ligament of the knee: a case report. PM R 2014;6(9):S279–80.
109. Kosy JD, Mandalia VI. Revisiting the anterolateral ligament of the knee. J Knee Surg 2016;29(7):571–9.
110. Feucht MJ, Zens M, Frosch K, et al. The anterolateral ligament of the knee: anatomy, biomechanics, and clinical implications. Curr Orthop Pract 2016;27(3):247–53.
111. Van dyck P, De smet E, Lambrecht V, et al. The anterolateral ligament of the knee: what the radiologist needs to know. Semin Musculoskelet Radiol 2016; 20(1):26–32.
112. Roessler PP, Schüttler KF, Heyse TJ, et al. The anterolateral ligament (ALL) and its role in rotational extra-articular stability of the knee joint: a review of anatomy and surgical concepts. Arch Orthop Trauma Surg 2016;136(3):305–13.

113. Bonasia DE, D'amelio A, Pellegrino P, et al. Anterolateral ligament of the knee: back to the future in anterior cruciate ligament reconstruction. Orthop Rev (Pavia) 2015;7(2):5773.
114. Cavaignac E, Ancelin D, Chiron P, et al. Historical perspective on the "discovery" of the anterolateral ligament of the knee. Knee Surg Sports Traumatol Arthrosc 2016;25(4):991–6.
115. Guenther D, Griffith C, Lesniak B, et al. Anterolateral rotatory instability of the knee. Knee Surg Sports Traumatol Arthrosc 2015;23(10):2909–17.

Moving?

Make sure your subscription moves with you!

To notify us of your new address, find your **Clinics Account Number** (located on your mailing label above your name), and contact customer service at:

Email: journalscustomerservice-usa@elsevier.com

800-654-2452 (subscribers in the U.S. & Canada)
314-447-8871 (subscribers outside of the U.S. & Canada)

Fax number: 314-447-8029

Elsevier Health Sciences Division
Subscription Customer Service
3251 Riverport Lane
Maryland Heights, MO 63043

*To ensure uninterrupted delivery of your subscription, please notify us at least 4 weeks in advance of move.